Living with Parkinson's Disease

Edited by
David Belgum

Hamilton Books
A member of
The Rowman & Littlefield Publishing Group
Lanham • Boulder • New York • Toronto • Plymouth, UK

Copyright © 2008 by
Hamilton Books
4501 Forbes Boulevard
Suite 200
Lanham, Maryland 20706
Hamilton Books Acquisitions Department (301) 459-3366

Estover Road
Plymouth PL6 7PY
United Kingdom

Library of Congress Control Number: 2007934989
ISBN-13: 978-0-7618-3861-6 (paperback : alk. paper)
ISBN-10: 0-7618-3861-9 (paperback : alk. paper)

∞™ The paper used in this publication meets the minimum
requirements of American National Standard for Information
Sciences—Permanence of Paper for Printed Library Materials,
ANSI Z39.48—1992

Contents

Preface   vii

INTRODUCTION   1

The Journey: Parkinson's Disease   3
Mary G. Baker, president, European Parkinson's Disease
Association and *Lizzie Graham*, project manager

The Shaking Palsy   13
Ian Maclean Smith, M.D., Emeritus Professor, Department of
Internal Medicine, University of Iowa Hospitals and Clinics

Part I

Legs   19
Stanley Elder

Say Hooray!!!   20
Sam Hahn

My World is Different Now   21
Pat Healy

It's a Long Way Down and Back   22
Sam Hahn

My New Canoeing Partner: Parkinson's   25
Bill Lyons

Running as Metaphor: A Personal Essay   27
Bob McCown

My Reflections   29
  David Good

Description of my Condition/Disability   31
  David Good

Choices   32
  Bill Lyons

Mental Acuity Tests   34
  Bill Lyons

Skis   35
  Pat Healy

After Diagnosis—What?   36
  Pat Healy

I Have Such a Wonderful Life   39
  Earl Rose

Parkinson's Disease: There is Life Before Death   40
  Earl Rose

Walking Sticks/Canes   42
  Earl and Marilyn Rose

The Once and Future Caregiver   44
  Caryl Lyons

To Caryl—Caregiver   47
  Bill Lyons

Just Say "Thanks": A Prose Poem   48
  Bob McCown

Part II

Showing Respect Through Creative Interchange   51
  Bill Lyons

Trust or Distrust   54
  Otto Bauer

Beatitude   57
  Earl Rose

Writing From Prison   58
  David Belgum

The Borderline Between Interpretation and Confidentiality 59
  David Belgum

Loose Canoe 60
  Bill Lyons

Building a Canoe of My Own 62
  David Good

Three Pieces from Learning From the Lizard and Stories Told
Under the Sycamore Tree 65
  Sam Hahn

The Meaning of Suffering 69
  David Belgum

Contributors 83

Preface

It has been a pleasure editing this collection of writings because they comprise a great variety of vocations and writing styles. There are essays, poetry, humor, etc. This is a frank sharing of what it means to have one's life touched by Parkinson's disease. Those who are primary clients help those who may be experiencing the beginning symptoms for the first time. They are not as alone as they had thought.

A person who has a health problem needs to be accepting, or as Alcoholics Anonymous members say, "To change what can be changed, to accept things that cannot be changed, and the wisdom to know the difference."

Our volume is divided into three parts. The introduction presents two previously published works on Parkinson's disease, one by a retired professor of internal medicine and the other by the president of the European Parkinson's Disease Association. Part I contains pieces about the experiences of Parkinson's patients and their caregivers. Part II consists of more general reflections about life that were also written by the members of our group.

Our writers group would be pleased if others experiment with other methods of sharing and caring. Speaking of caring, you will notice that caregivers are also included because their lives are touched by this disease in various ways. If you should wish to respond to this writing in one way or another, you may do so by writing to Kathie Belgum (spouse):

Kathie Belgum
104 Sunset Street
Iowa City, Iowa 52246

INTRODUCTION

The Journey: Parkinson's Disease[1]

Mary G. Baker, *President, European Parkinson's Disease Association* and Lizzie Graham, *Project Manager*

INTRODUCTION

To receive a diagnosis of a chronic neurological illness is the beginning of a long journey into the unknown—a journey that may begin in hope, pass through periods of elation and frustration, and finally end in acceptance and resignation. We would like you to come with us part of the way along the journey of Parkinson's disease, seen from the point of view of those who are compelled to make it—the patients and their carers.

THE MAP

When we begin any journey, we need a map. We need to pack and prepare for the journey. We need to know what to expect along the way. The telling of the diagnosis and the explanation of the disease and its treatment form just such a map. And, like the maps of the medieval world, the map of Parkinson's disease is full of unknown territories and nameless threats. Small wonder that the telling of the diagnosis is so difficult. But it is so important and is one of the things that patients repeatedly say could be done better.

People begin the journey with different knowledge and different ways of accepting the disease. The telling must be adjusted to take account of education, intelligence, and cultural background. Not all patients will be well educated, not all will be able to read, and not all will be able to speak well the language of the country in which they are living.

Many patients and their families will have misconceptions about Parkinson's disease that need to be dealt with. One of the best ways to explore the meaning of the diagnosis is to ask patients: "What do you know about Parkinson's disease?" and "What do you want to know?" Among the most common questions are: "Will I die?" "Will I be able to work?" "What will I tell the children?" Then, there are other questions that may not be voiced: "Who will care for me when I can no longer care for myself?" "What will this disease do to my relationships?" Let's look at some of the areas that need to be dealt with if patients are to be able to set out on their journey properly prepared.

WHERE THE MAP STARTS AND ENDS

The average age for developing Parkinson's disease is around 65, although up to one in 10 people with the disease develop it in their 40s or 50s. Globally, Parkinson's disease affects 6.3 million people, with one in 10 people receiving a diagnosis before age 50 (www.epda.eu.com).

The symptoms usually appear slowly and develop gradually and in no particular order. It is important to remember that everyone with Parkinson's disease is different and may have a different collection of symptoms and response to treatment from another person with the same diagnosis. The symptoms may take years to progress to a point where they cause major problems, and when they do, many of these symptoms can be treated.

But telling a patient that Parkinson's disease is treatable and leaving him or her with the impression that this means "curable" will do a great disservice to the patient. Honesty is essential—it does not have to be brutal. Although Parkinson's disease has no cure, it is the only neurodegenerative disorder with a range of medical and neurosurgical treatments that substantially reduce symptoms. Having said that, patients need to know that these treatments sometimes lead to disappointment and may have side effects in the long term that prove more troublesome than the disease.

Professionals Who Can Help with the Management of Parkinson's Disease

- General practitioner
- Neurologist
- Gerontologist
- Psychologist
- Nurse specialist
- Occupational therapist
- Physiotherapist
- Dietician

- Speech and language therapist
- Pharmacist
- Social worker
- Chiropodist

Parkinson's disease by itself does not directly cause people to die. With the treatments now available, life expectancy for someone with Parkinson's disease is fairly normal. However, for people who are seriously disabled (usually those who have had the disease for many years), their general physical and mental condition can either cause or exacerbate other illnesses and so contribute to the final cause of death.

The period of adjustment to the diagnosis will vary—in some cases, it may take years for people to come to terms with their situation, during which time everyone in the family will suffer and relationships will change. Ultimately, each patient will make his or her own way along the journey, but hopefully, he or she will not have to make it alone.

TRAVELING COMPANIONS

The patients and carers who embark on the journey should be aware from the outset that they do not have to travel alone. Neither should the doctor be the only person who is there to help them carry their physical and emotional baggage. The burden is much better shared among a multidisciplinary team.

The journey involves not only the patient and professionals but also partners, family, and friends. It is a mistake, however, to assume that suffering always brings people together—sometimes it does not. Not everyone is sustained by happy and loving relationships. A rocky relationship is unlikely to be saved by the crushing blow of chronic incurable illness.

European Parkinson's Disease Association and World Health Organization: Charter of Rights for People with Parkinson's Disease

People with Parkinson's have the right to:

- Be referred to a doctor with a special interest in Parkinson's
- Receive an accurate diagnosis
- Have access to support services
- Receive continuous care and
- Take part in managing the illness.

Declared on this day the 11th Day of April 1997 (cited from www.epda.eu).

To put it bluntly, not everyone asked to join the journey will want to go. Some will, with great sadness, put down their packs and refuse to go on, either at the start or at some point along the way. This is their right, and we, as professionals should not assume that all partners and families are capable of seeing the journey through.

Parkinson's disease changes relationships between couples in many ways. Not all couples are well equipped to cope; some patients find it very hard to be dependent on their partner, and some partners feel guilty about not wanting to be the main carer. Loss of self esteem, along with the physical problems of general fatigue, shaking, muscle stiffness, and dribbling may lead to sexual difficulties, as will erectile problems. Parkinson's disease may also worsen or be worsened by problems with menstruation, contraception, pregnancy, and the menopause. Yet this is an area that receives scant attention. More practical advice is needed on how to cope with the difficulties from day to day, and more research is also needed—for example, into the interactions of antiparkinsonian medications with the menstrual cycle, with oral contraceptives, and with hormone replacement therapy. Patients rarely voice these concerns spontaneously and may need to be asked sensitively about them.

Hugs and cuddles may be physically difficult for patients with Parkinson's disease to give and receive. This may be particularly difficult to understand for and even be frightening to younger children in the family, who don't know what to make of an impassive face and confusing body language. Generally, children handle honesty far better than deceit, and research shows that children are usually relieved to be told that their mother's or father's strangeness is caused by Parkinson's disease.

The adult offspring of people with Parkinson's disease may have to face the responsibilities of caring for a disabled parent and have to make painful decisions about their own plans for the future and about who will care for their parent.

WHAT TRAVELERS NEED ALONG THE WAY

Patients tell us that there are five things that they need to help them to live better with Parkinson's disease. They need to be referred to a doctor with a special interest in this disease. They need a better telling of the diagnosis. They need access to the multidisciplinary team. They need continuity of care, and they need to participate in the management of their own illness.

The European Parkinson's Disease Association, in collaboration with the World Health Organization, developed these five principles into a "charter" for people with Parkinson's disease, launched in London on the first World Parkinson's Disease Day, 11 April 1997. This charter has been signed and supported by global organisations for Parkinson's disease and by well known celebrities.

Doctors are the chroniclers of the journey. We hope that close collaborations will help us to develop models of integrated care that will draw together the best in modern medical practice, using all the strengths of the multidisciplinary team and involving the patients themselves.

For example, doctors should not forget that many patients value physical therapy as much as, if not more than, medication, to help them move and remain active. The Association of Physiotherapists in Parkinson's Disease Europe has developed guidelines for physiotherapy practice in Parkinson's disease, following two Cochrane systematic reviews of physiotherapy and Parkinson's disease, and these are available on the internet (http://appde.unn.ac.uk).

Occupational therapy can also teach patients ways to adapt to their symptoms and continue to do the activities that are important to them. Speech and language therapy may be a great help too, not only for voice training but also to improve and maintain swallowing and to avoid subsequent problems such as choking, undernutrition, and pneumonia.

Health professionals may also find it hard to share their patients' enthusiasm for complementary or alternative therapies. Some of these may have some benefit, even if it is largely psychological. Although it is clearly difficult for health professionals to endorse treatments they do not believe in, there is no reason why they should not take a tolerant and accepting attitude towards measures such as meditation, aromatherapy, yoga, the Alexander technique, osteopathy, and so on. If patients feel better, for any reason, we can only be grateful.

A specialist nurse is often the best person to draw together the strands of multidisciplinary care and to be the key contact for patients and caregivers, providing the continuity of care those patients have identified as one of their primary needs.

TRAVELING ALONE

One of the hardest things to face in Parkinson's disease is the loss of independence and a sense of isolation or exclusion from normal life. Doctors sometimes advise younger patients to give up work, but this is not a step that should be taken lightly or without proper assessment and support from occupational health services (if available). The impact on the family is not confined to the loss of earnings. The loss of self esteem, the dashing of expectations, and the stress of changing family roles can erode relationships. Not everyone has rich reserves of self worth, or a lively circle of friends and acquaintances, to help them feel that there is a life worth living beyond work. Isolation is often compounded by the patient's introspection and gradual withdrawal from the world beyond the narrow confines of their disease.

Another aspect that patients often mention is having to give up driving—the practical and psychological consequences of depending on others are hard to take. But many people with Parkinson's disease can, and do, continue to drive for many years after the diagnosis, if supported by their doctor. However, in the United Kingdom and many other countries patients have a legal obligation to inform the Driver and Vehicle Licensing Agency (or its local equivalent) of their diagnosis and may need to have a medical examination or take a driving test.

LOSING THE PATH

Even if the people who set out are well prepared and have a helpful team of guides and supporters the journey will never be easy. For most patients the journey, after the initial shock of the diagnosis, moves into sunlight. There may be a honeymoon period in which treatment is working well and other people, at work and socially, are unaware of the illness. Slowly, the landscape of the disease changes. The journey becomes dark and difficult, and often lonely. The travelers may lose their way or follow false trails. The dragons of dyskinesia and depression appear, to be fought again and again.

Patient's Story

Terry and I had reached the point in our lives when we were established in a nice home, we were financially secure, and life was looking good for our family. But life has the knack of taking you by surprise, and suddenly our lives were turned upside down by a series of events which started with Terry being diagnosed with Parkinson's. Having no knowledge of Parkinson's or any understanding of the condition, I was filled with fear of what the future held for us all. I was utterly convinced that within six months he would be confined to a wheelchair. Then two months later I was diagnosed with cervical cancer and was told that I would have to have a hysterectomy.

I felt there was no one I could turn to, so I shelved any fears I had about me. All I needed was to find out all I could about Parkinson's, so I went to the public library and the information I found there frightened me even more. At night I would lie awake watching Terry to see if his tremor had worsened or spread to another part of his body. My children seemed unable to accept that their father had Parkinson's, which stopped me from discussing it with them, and I felt so isolated. Terry, being Terry, continued to try to live his life as he always had. He had always been the "strong" one, the protector, the provider. But now I felt he was not the same and that he needed my protection. In a few short months, our roles, which had always been secure and constant, had changed.

The telling of a diagnosis whether it be Parkinson's or cancer is crucial. We, the patients, rely on the expertise of the medical profession. If they misdiagnose an illness it can have a catastrophic effect on our lives. We also need easily accessible and accurate information to help us to adjust to the many changes that we have to face.

Our lives have changed, and so have we. I have become more assertive and self assured, and have found strengths within myself which I did not know existed. On reflection, I wonder whether I have made a mistake by taking too much of the burden on to my own shoulders. I honestly feel that people refuse to discuss the most serious problems in their lives at a time when you should express your true feelings. But we rarely do so, as we are frightened to break down and embarrass ourselves as well as our families and friends. Because of my fear I felt a strong need to protect Terry, but perhaps by my actions, I have inadvertently undermined his self confidence. He is after all still Terry, who just happens to have Parkinson's.

Depression is one of the commonest problems encountered in Parkinson's disease and is under-recognised and under-researched. One of the biggest surveys into quality of life, the Global Parkinson's Disease Survey (GPDS), carried out in seven countries in 1998–1999, identified that depression reduced quality of life considerably. Half of the people surveyed were depressed, but only 1% had reported this as a problem. It is not clear whether the disease itself causes depression or whether depression is a reaction to the situation in which the patient finds himself or herself. Depression is an equally common problem for carers, although those who feel guilty at not being able to cope may conceal it.

Patients also encounter other problems as the disease progresses: nausea, hot sweats, dilated pupils, nightmares and hallucinations, confusion, and memory loss. Some of these may be due to the disease, others to the side effects of the medication. Whatever the cause, the patient is assailed by the terrifying feeling of being out of control. Instead the disease, or its treatment, is controlling him or her.

Please, as doctors, listen to what your patients have to tell you about medical treatment. The patient's perception of overdose or inadequate dosing may be quite different from your own. People may vary widely in the degree of symptoms that they are willing to tolerate. Consultation, not confrontation, is the way to achieve compliance and concordance. Remember that one of the five things that the patient needs most is to take some of the responsibility for their own management.

TRAVELER'S TALES

Often patients and caregivers learn new ways of coping with Parkinson's disease by sharing experiences with others in the same position (see patient's story). This is where the Parkinson's disease organizations come in, such as the European Parkinson's Disease Association.

JOURNEY'S END

Not everyone starts the journey from the same point, in terms of knowledge and expectations. Better telling of the diagnosis is needed. Patients need clear maps and signposts along their journey, to help them cope with treatment; physical problems; the world of work, family, and relationships; and the depression they may encounter along the way. Patients do not undertake their journey alone, but not every member of their family may be willing or able to travel with them. Doctors do not have to carry all the burden of supporting the patients—the multidisciplinary team and patients' organizations are there to help.

European Parkinson's Disease Association

The European Parkinson's Disease Association was formed in Munich in 1992 with a membership of nine European organizations for Parkinson's patients, and its membership has since increased to 35, with nine associate members including the Movement Disorder Society, the Association of Physiotherapists in Parkinson's Disease Europe, the European Federation of Neurological Associations, and the Tremor Foundation. The association's purpose is to develop a dialogue between science and society and to effect change by shaping European policy and education, resulting in improved quality of life for people with Parkinson's disease. The association is committed to ensuring that people with Parkinson's disease, their families, and their friends do not have to make the journey alone but have the best possible support from the healthcare professions, from the social and welfare agencies, and from each other.

The association is a non-political, non-religious, and non-profit making organization concerned with the health and welfare of people living with Parkinson's disease and their families. It has provided an important forum to work in collaboration with international organizations, both patient and neurological. These include the European Commission, the World Health Organization, the World Federation of Neurology, and the pharmaceutical industry. This partnership has enabled the development of research projects into quality of life issues, production of validated information on Parkinson's disease, its medication and how to manage the complexities of its management, and biannual conferences for multidisciplinary teams and people of any age with Parkinson's disease.

The right information is crucial for any journey to be successful; without it, people end up going in the wrong direction. The European Parkinson's Disease Association is very well aware how important it is to provide validated information, for people to be able to access this and to make their own choices as to whether or not to use it. The association's website, www.epda.eu.com has been developed to provide such information and include information not only about Parkinson's disease, its management and medication, but also on magazines and on books written by people with Parkinson's disease and professionals, and links to other websites about holidays and organizations that could be of help.

Further Reading for Patients, Caregivers, and Doctors

A series of six information leaflets for patients, produced in 2004, is a helpful and accurate resource for people with Parkinson's, their families, and healthcare professionals. To date they have been translated into eight languages, with more translations planned throughout the year—www.epda.eu.com.

Anderson, S. *Health is between your ears. Living with a chronic disease.* Hornslet, Denmark, Parkinson Info, 2002. This book, by a Danish psychologist diagnosed in 1989, was written for people with Parkinson's and their families, to regain optimism, and to show that despite the disease, life can still be good—www.epda.eu.com.

Aho, K. *Parkinson's disease: my constant companion a neurologist's experiences as a patient.* Brussels: European Parkinson's Disease Association, 2002. Successful treatment of Parkinson's disease is an art. In addition to a good doctor-patient relationship, the patient's own activity and initiative have a central role. Alongside medical treatment, the right type of nutrition often brings added help.

Baker, MG, Marsden, CD, Oxtoby, M, Williams, A, Moore, L, Woodroffe, D, et al. *Parkinson's at your fingertips.* 2nd ed. London: Class Publishing 1999.

Clear and helpful information on Parkinson's, written in a very accessible question and answer format—www.parkinsons.org.uk.

Parkinson's Disease Society. *Parkinson's aware in primary care*. London: PDS, 2003. Written mainly by general practitioners, for general practitioners and the wider primary care team, this is a guide for the best management of Parkinson's disease. As well as information on Parkinson's and the drug treatment available, the leaflet gives guidelines on procedure at four key stages: diagnosis, maintenance, complex and palliative —www.parkinsons.org.uk/ shared_asp_files/uploadedfiles/{ 31E42B83-775B-414F-B3C4-8708E9DC 0B2C}_PDAware PrimaryCareSept03.pdf.

Infopark (www.infopark.uwcm.ac.uk)—brought together academics, clinicians, and user groups to explore the information needs of older people with disabilities in Europe. The research project involved partners from the United Kingdom, Spain, Portugal, Estonia, Germany, Greece, and Finland. Information sheets in six languages on Parkinson's disease have been developed based on the results of patients', carers', and professionals' concerns.

www.parkinsonpoly.com—The need for education and information for people with Parkinson's disease and their carers has been the driving force behind this innovative program, which uses the web and visual mnemonics. In 2004, it is being translated into many languages.

www.besttreatments.co.uk—Has brought together the best research about Parkinson's disease and weighed up the evidence about how to treat it. People with Parkinson's disease can use the information to talk with their doctor and decide which treatments are best for them.

NOTE

1. Reprinted with permission of the BMJ Publishing Group. Also available on-line at: http://bmj.bmjjournals.com/cgi/content/full/329/7466/611

The Shaking Palsy[1]

Ian Maclean Smith, M.D., *Emeritus Professor,*
Department of Internal Medicine,
University of Iowa Hospitals and Clinics

As a young intern, I had eight patients with Parkinson's disease in the chronic part of my 60-bed ward. There were no effective drugs available then to slow down the crippling effect of the disease and my inability to help them frustrated me.

Sir James Parkinson, in 1817, first described many of the typical symptoms: the tremor or shaking, loss of muscular power, and the way the body bends forward while walking, sometimes passing from a walking to a running pace to avoid falling.

A doctor determines whether or not patients have Parkinson's disease without taking any blood tests. Doctors look for stooped posture, stiffness and slowness of movement, fixed facial expression, and four per second rhythmic tremor of the hands.

It is the tremor that most often brings patients to the doctor's office. This is usually of the hands, but a woman I saw recently only had tremor of the chin. This is a "resting tremor" because it typically happens when the patient's hands are idle. Some people develop a tremor that is completely unrelated to Parkinson's disease, benign hereditary tremor. It happens when people are doing something, not at rest. It is not serious and can be treated.

Parkinson's disease is due to nerve cell loss in the substantial nigra (literally the black stuff) of the mid brain. It can be seen with the naked eye and it contains dopamine, which is essential for the control of movement. Why the cells in the substantial nigra die and stop making dopamine is unknown, but this area can be poisoned by carbon monoxide, manganese, a virus as in the epidemic of von Economo's encephalitis of 1918 to 1925, or a "street" drug chemical MPTP. This is a by-product of the street production of Demerol and astonished its producer and some friends by almost completely paralyzing them after intravenous injection. Similar chemicals are being looked for as environmental insults which might be a cause of Parkinsonism. Other causes of Parkinson-like disease should be mentioned. Namely, punch drunkenness, like Mohammed Ali, or the necessary use or overuse of phenothiazine drugs, such as chlorpromazine used as major tranquilizers.

Dopamine will not enter the central nervous system, however, a mirror image precursor, levodopa, will. Combined with an anti-enzyme to prevent loss of active drug it becomes a combination drug called Carbidopa. Bromocriptin (trade name Parlodel) from the wheat rust ergot, chemically mimics the effect of dopamine and can be added. Other drugs with usefulness in the disease are propranalol, several anticholinergics, and the anti-influenza drug, amantadine. Use of sinus and the common cold medicines can seriously disrupt treatment. Even the most carefully managed drug program can only help to slow the progress of this presently incurable disease. A new breakthrough has been the prevention of advancement of the disease with Deprenyl, under active research study at present.

Good management requires cooperation between the physician, the patient, and the patient's relatives. In advanced cases, activity must be maintained and the patient must be given every assistance, such as an electric razor, shoes without laces, and clothing with velcro closures. Since patients may be capable of much more independence one time than the next, it is important that families realize that the patient is not "faking" weakness or inability.

Another experimental approach to the treatment of Parkinsonism is to try to put dopamine forming human tissue in the brain. Transplantation of adrenal tissue has been unsuccessful but the transplantation of fetal brain tissue has caused a small number of patients to live more independently with a 40% decrease in the need for drugs and an increase in their daily activities, leading to cautious optimism about a possible treatment for the future.

There are three important complications of Parkinsonism. One-third of advanced disease patients develop dementia and half of them develop depression. The depression is treatable with the usual anti-depressive drugs. Parkinson's may be complicated by the so-called on-off phenomenon where the patient abruptly alternates between marked immobility and mobility with added involuntary movements which is very hard to manage.

In 1944, I used to treat my Parkinsonism patients with tincture of stramonium (from jimsonweed) which was the only drug that we had. After a week's treatment, I would tell my chief that I was curing them. "Anecdotal research, Smith. Anecdotal research will lead you astray," he commented. In the decades from 1960 onwards, very sophisticated research has been done on Parkinson's disease and a successful program of drugs, exercise, and medical supervision can make it possible to live longer with a higher quality of life despite this previously totally disabling disease.

NOTE

1. Reprinted with permission of the author. Also available on-line at: http://lib .cpums.edu.cn/jiepou/tupu/atlas/www.vh.org/adult/patient/internalmedicine/aba30/ 1993/parkin.html

Part I

Legs

Stanley Elder

They carried me down a country road
to a country school

They carried me across a high school
basketball court and football field

They carried me into the belly of a
B-17 bomber in wartime

They carried me to meet
my bride at the altar

They carried me across farmlands
awakening with green

They carried me up a ladder
to build our retirement home

Now they have betrayed me:
I have Parkinson's.

Say Hooray!!!

Sam Hahn

These crazy legs don't work no more
They've kind of gone to jerkin
They're sorta glued down most every day
Except when the medicine is workin

My writin also is mostly bad
The letters are kind of smallish
I need to magnify what I read
And see there's no squish to dish

And then there's constipation too,
Once a month I move them
The Power Pudding helped a lot
Prune juice don't even cure 'em

My hands may work part of the time
At least they let me drive yet
If pressure mounts they fumble more
And more when I stew and fret

Bed time means lying like a board
I need a hoist to turn me
A bedside pot is needed now
I face more loss of dignity

Saliva drips from off my chin
Drooling is one of the symptoms
What more can I do to shut it off?
Maybe hide some place in the catacombs

So what is your story of Parkinson's?
Don't worry there's help on the way
By the time we're 100 we'll be fixed up
So today as you pray say HOORAY!!!

My World is Different Now

Pat Healy

The world is full of beauty,
I look at life differently now,
I appreciate Mother Nature more,
I express myself more freely,
I give more than I receive,
I have learned to be patient,
I am willing to listen.
I am thankful for each day anew.
I plunge forward on this journey.
To remain strong,
I desire to be healthy.
I will stand up and fight for my life.
I will pray for others in their journeys.
I will be persistent in seeking a cure.
I stand tall for all I believe.
I believe in miracles,
I believe in angels,
I believe I am surrounded by the light.
I believe in healing and in a world of peace.
May God keep you in his palm,
May God protect from wind and rain,
and other acts of Mother Nature.
May you find everlasting peace
and walk with God's loving hands.
Fill your life with prayer,
Life is so fragile.

It's a Long Way Down and Back

Sam Hahn

Why would a seventy-four-year-old geezer attempt to walk to the bottom of the Grand Canyon? Even our St. Mark's Church found it significant enough to include a notation in its newsletter. That place is deep and wide. How deep? The highest point is about 9,000 feet above sea level. The river at the base of the canyon is 1,850 feet above sea level. So it is more than a mile down from the lower parts of the rim.

The North Rim of the canyon rises about 1,200 feet higher than the South Rim. The North Rim is at such a high level, that snow melt is much later, and the North Rim does not open until mid May. So hiking generally goes from the South rim, most going down the South Kaibob trail, about eight miles long. We returned by the Bright Angel Trail, a longer but more gradual trail, nearly ten miles long.

My hike into the Canyon began at the Kaibob Trail Head which is east of the main park headquarters. There were nine hikers in our group, each carrying a backpack ranging in weight from ten to twenty-five pounds. An adequate water supply is a must, but one mistake many hikers make is to carry too many things. Some of necessity even carried their sleeping bag. My backpack, including water, food, a change of clothes and cameras, weighed fifteen pounds.

About three-fourths mile down the Kaibob Trail we came to the appropriately named, "Ooh Aah Point."; a place where a whole new magnificent array of canyon color is visible, and an ideal place to be at sunset. I did real well on the hike down. Legs didn't bother me, as is often the case in the steep downhill hike, and I kept ahead of most of our group. I communicated with daughter Eunice on her walkie-talkie. There is a dark tunnel when the bottom is reached that leads to a sturdy secure bridge over the Colorado River. By that time I was getting tired and greatly relieved to come to Phantom Ranch, a variety of buildings made from stone and logs including small dormitories with sleeping room for ten on bunk beds, including shower. Also a dining hall seating about fifty, some park business buildings, and a large tent and sleeping bag area, some sheltered by a roof.

With the evening approaching, the sinking sun intensifies the colors of the canyon walls, now reaching and reaching a mile almost straight up. At its widest point the canyon is eighteen miles wide. I was fortunate enough to secure a sleeping bed in one of the dorms. Close by was the dining hall where we were served generous helpings of stew and corn bread topped off with generous servings of chocolate cake. Not a bargain. The evening meal was $21.07, noon sack lunch was $9.59, bunk bed lodging was $28.00 each night. We hiked in on Thursday April 14th, stayed there the 15th and hiked out on the 16th.

Eunice didn't think old Dad should sit around on Friday, so she led me on another trail toward the North Rim, about three miles total, but a steep climb and again more of the canyon's splendor was visible. The rangers night time presentation was on the value and splendor of the night. Above us the moon and the stars were more visible than they are in any city.

I also went to the beach along the Colorado River, close to where Bright Angel stream empties into the Colorado. Bright Angel was running at bank full, in places a raging stream as the snow areas high up were melting. To my disappointment no bathing beauties were there, in fact no one was at the beach. I stuck my feet into the frigid water and realized why no one was there. Tied to the beach were two large rubber raft boats for rafting the Colorado. They get on far up the river where the canyon is shallow, and leave for downstream where it is accessible without the long canyon walk.

Friday morning we were up early for 5:00 A.M. breakfast. And that also was a large meal. We were on the Bright Angel trail before 7:00 A.M. with ten miles of hiking ahead. Uphill all the way. Again the weather for hiking was ideal. At the ranch the highs reached eighty-eight. On the South Rim the temperature was sixty-six. Compared to the bridge we crossed the Colorado on coming into the ranch, as we returned across the river the bridge was unstable and small, not used for mule trains. Whenever we did meet a mule train we gave them the trail. They are very sure footed. Part time they carried people; part time they carried supplies. Virtually everything is brought in by mule (one reason the food at the ranch is so expensive). About the only time helicopters are used is to evacuate someone with a medical problem.

My Parkinson's medication did its work and I was able to keep going. The hike out took about eleven hours. At least an hour of that time was spent for breaks, lunch, and rest time. There is only one rest room on the way down; going back there are water and facilities at the China Garden area about half way out. We had our lunch there. Then, with three miles to go, we came to another restroom stop, and with one and a half miles to go there is another.

A good Samaritan, Phil Mennenoh, my son-in-law, came to our rescue at the China Garden, and carried backpacks for two of the girls. By that time they had blisters and greatly appreciated the help. By the grace of God I was able to continue to carry my pack all the way.

All along the trail there were multitudes of blooming spring flowers. There was time for picture taking, and some of them were incredibly large and colorful flowers.

In summary I want to include a statement by Stephen G. Maurer, author of seven books about the area:

> As you stand on either rim of the Grand Canyon peering down at a ribbon of water, it is as if you are standing outside the frame of a picture, observing. A trip down, however, is one of the ways you can experience the incredible scenery of the Grand Canyon.

My wife, Juanita, because of health conditions was unable to attempt the trip into the Canyon. She claims her enjoyment came from doing dusting of many, many native American Indian hand crafted items our daughter has collected. She also spent quality time with our Grand Dogs, Gus and Toby, loveable pets that even accompany the family to church every Sunday.

My New Canoeing Partner: Parkinson's

Bill Lyons

When I step into or out of a canoe, it helps if another person holds me from behind, by my belt. That's right. I bend over, they grab my belt and act like a crane, you know, for lifting big pieces of equipment from one place to another. In this case, the object being lifted, or at least assisted, is me. Without someone's hand around my belt, I am unsteady and feel as though I might topple over the canoe and into the lake. Have I toppled? No, not in that situation. But I have fallen often enough in other situations to be tired of falling and to try to avoid it.

Once I caught the toe of my slipper under the edge of a floor register. As I fell, I missed the square corners of several pieces of furniture. For my second adventure in space travel, I tripped on a piece of raised concrete driveway. I fell flat but hit my head first on the bumper of a car, a car new enough that the bumper was hard plastic instead of metal. My head hit the concrete more slowly than if the bumper had not been there. Someone brought an ice pack to keep down the swelling, and after twenty minutes I was okay. Another time, I was hustling to keep up with my two young granddaughters, didn't watch my feet carefully (I have partial vision), caught the toe of one shoe on a piece of concrete sidewalk that had been pushed up by a tree root, fell and jammed my glasses into my right cheek, near my eye, opening a cut that took eleven stitches to close. I had a black eye for a while, and later tried to assure the granddaughters, by telephone, that I was again a handsome grandfather whose face no longer looked like a mudball target. In the yard, as an experiment, I loaded two forty-pound bags of softener salt into the wheelbarrow and began to push it around the back of the house to the outside basement door. When the wheelbarrow tipped, I tried to keep it upright and was thrown to the ground, firmer than I remembered. Then inside, vacuuming, I caught my foot in the cord and fell on carpet, again bending my glasses and, this time, getting a forehead floor burn.

So, have I experienced toppling? Yes, enough to want not to fall into a canoe or even into a lake. Sometimes the "canoe crew" consists of one person, usually my wife, Caryl. Or, if we are canoeing with another couple, two or even three people. With this kind of help, I can be confident of my having a smooth move into and, later, out of the canoe.

Once in the boat, I can paddle a good long time before tiring. Where have we paddled since my "iffy" balance became a factor? 1) Lake MacBride, with its inlet streams on the east end, featuring blue herons, Canadian geese, red-winged blackbirds, muskrats, beaver, deer, and in the shallows, carp. 2) Big Lake, tucked in among lakes in the western Boundary Waters Canoe Area in northern Minnesota, with beaver, loons, and ducks, and 3) several connected lakes in northern Wisconsin, near Boulder Junction. In both Minnesota and Wisconsin, we rented a cabin with our friends David and Kerry Evans, stayed a week, and canoed. Welcome aboard to my new canoeing partner, Parkinson's. Let's paddle.

Running as Metaphor:
A Personal Essay

Bob McCown

In the 1970s in the United States running became a fad. Jim Fixx's book enti-
tled *Running* was a national best seller and marathon runners Frank Shorter and
Bill Rogers were often in the sports pages. *Runner's World*, a monthly maga-
zine devoted to the sport, zoomed in sales. Later the craze was satirized in the
movie, *Forrest Gump* (1994) starring Tom Hanks. With encouragement of a
friend, I began running, or "jogging" as some called it, in the spring of 1978. I
had participated in track in high school and college, but then I was a sprinter,
and now I would be a distance runner. My first workouts were on the grassy
fields of City Park in Iowa City. At the end of July on a hot Sunday evening my
friend and I ran our first road race. The five-mile course began in the front of
Old Capitol on the University of Iowa campus in downtown Iowa City and ran
through City Park, Manville Heights, and back to the Old Capitol. At the beginning of the race, I was amazed by the speed of the elite runners and I realized that a good deal of training would be necessary to bring me to that level. I
was exhilarated by the experience and I knew that I would be running more
races. By fall I completed a half marathon, 13.1 miles, in a respectable time.

At some point in my early days of training my daughter gave me a Nike tee-
shirt picturing a landscape with a lone runner bearing the caption "There is no
finish line." I took this adage as an aphorism: I would keep running for the rest
of my life. In 1979 I set a goal of running a marathon, 26.1 miles, and I un-
dertook to prepare physically. During the spring and summer I ran a number
of races of varying length, always trying to improve my speed and endurance.
I found that I relished the competition and by the late summer I was running
as much as 75 miles a week. On November 4, 1979, I completed the Iowa City
MS Marathon in just over three hours, a few weeks short of my fortieth birth-
day. I still consider this race as one of the high points of my personal life.

Perhaps the part of running that I enjoyed the most was the camaraderie of the runners. A local sporting goods store was the Mecca for runners in the late 1970s and early 1980s. In addition to selling running shoes and other paraphernalia, the staff of the store organized fun runs and training runs. There was usually a small entry fee and one of the rewards was the obligatory tee-shirt. When a whole drawer in our chest of drawers became filled with running tee-shirts, I gave the shirts to Goodwill. My wife now regrets not using them to make a quilt. I came to know some of the other runners, people that I would not meet in my professional life. I ran with geologists, social workers, poets, journalists, physicians, and others. Races were also a social event for families. Quite often we would carpool to runs in Cedar Rapids and Davenport. Later there was a running club, the Iowa City Striders. For a time I was the secretary for the group.

Over the next thirteen years I continued to run even when I was attending professional meetings or on business trips. I have good memories of running in such cities as Baltimore, New Orleans, Chicago, Providence, Los Angeles, Austin, Nashville, Saint Louis, and Washington D.C. Because of the increasing demands on my professional life, I ran less as the years passed quickly. Still, by 1989 I ran three or four days a week, My last competition was on October 14, 1984, at the Iowa City Hospice Race where I ran 3.1 miles in 17.37 minutes for first place in the 40- to 49-year-old category

In the spring and summer of 1992 I began to notice that on evening runs my left arm did not swing and at some point my left leg stiffened and I was unable to run. After walking a block or two, I could resume running again. I consulted my family practice physician and he volunteered to run with me to observe the condition. He prescribed some exercises with weights as a possible remedy and followed up by my having a CAT scan to rule out a brain tumor. Because symptoms continued I was referred to the Neurology Department at the University of Iowa Hospitals and Clinics. There I was diagnosed with Parkinson's Disease and put under the care of a specialist. My motto had not come true; there was a finish line after all. My last run was in the countryside near Fargo, North Dakota, while on a family visit.

Being unable to run any more did not mean that I abandoned exercise. I had always enjoyed walking and I had made it a practice to walk to and from work five days a week, no matter what the weather. The distance was about two miles one way. I also continued stretching exercises and the use of weights. In these activities, my loving wife stressed that keeping fit improves the quality of life. After my retirement from work at the end of 2001, I had more time for such exercise.

While I have crossed the finish line in running, I have many more lines to cross before the end of the course that may present even greater challenges for me.

My Reflections

David Good

We're always in transition, moving in a direction. I'm not going to particularly write about my perspective looking back, a historical perspective, but rather about what I'm thinking now.

I have always been independent. Now I find myself having to rely on others to assist me. I am confined to a smaller space geographically as I can't get in my car and drive somewhere. I can go on my bike but it isn't the same. When it's night or too cold to ride my bike, my friends or my wife take me to pottery or coffee with my former law partners or to Harmony Hawks chorus practice.

Because I am more dependent I have less freedom and am also more accountable. I choose to be more accountable because people care about me. To help my wife, whenever I leave home I carry my cell phone and have it on so she can call and know I'm "okay."

When I was a child, I was told to "stop, look, and listen" at street and railroad crossings. When I was more independent, my thinking was more automatic and so were my responses. I didn't have to actually stop, look and listen. Now I find I am consciously stopping to not only look and listen but also to think. I wish to retain as much of my independence as I can so I find I have to be more thoughtful before I take action. Intentionally I think slower to make sure I cover the bases of safety and appropriateness. I've always been safety conscious and have no reason to believe I haven't always been appropriate but now I am more thoughtful about it.

It feels that sometimes there are people who know me who don't know what to say to me or don't want to interact with me anymore. I always used to freely reach out to others. Before I didn't have to think about reaching out. Now my brain slows me down. I may have five, ten or thirty things going in my brain but my brain gets filled up and it locks up. So I know the person but I can't get their name out. It's hard to communicate that to the other person. Communication is impeded and that's a problem.

Since I now don't automatically reach out and seem more hesitant, some people I've known before my condition was diagnosed may not know how to react to the change or handle the difference. I have feelings because I have difficulty being able to start conversations. Others may have feelings also. We don't talk about feelings because it doesn't flow within the course of conversation. Recently I have been trying to take as much responsibility as I can for initiating talk and being social, more so than I did after my condition was first diagnosed. I am aware that it takes more energy.

It feels like there is only so much space in my brain at any one time. I can't switch tracks as fast or put words out like I used to be able to do.

I still feel able to make myself happy and not withstanding the changes I've noted with friendships, I enjoy almost everyone I meet and I don't worry much about the people who don't seem to know what to say to me.

I have found that many people have come into my life. I have met people I may not have met if I didn't have this condition as I might not be doing some of the things I am doing now. These people are a blessing. They relate to me as I am now, not as I was before this condition developed. They didn't know me before.

Having retired due to this disability and no longer having a job is a loss and a gift. I miss the routine of a daily job and having contact and conversation with colleagues daily. But now I really like the time I have to enjoy the things of life and people and not to be in a rush like I was when I worked. I remember the day that I was on the trail around Cedar Lake and at my leisure could enjoy watching the birds hatch and chirp. I have time to watch the bugs on trees and all the great things of nature.

I've been able to do new things because I now have time. I go to pottery class on Wednesday mornings at Ambrose Recreation Center, I struggle with it to some degree, but I think I might be getting better. It's been a challenge. I joined the Harmony Hawks chorus. It has been and always is great. I started going to the YMCA to swim. There are people in all these places who have been very helpful and have enhanced my life. They offer to help and assist me. I am very thankful for them and how they've helped me be able to participate even though I have this condition or disability.

P.S. I love my kayak. I think it's the safest thing on the water. It feels like home.

Description of My Condition/Disability

David Good

My condition is called posterior cortical atrophy. It is pretty rare. Mayo Clinic has diagnosed only sixty-eight cases since 1988. This condition means that the part of my brain that processes what I see has atrophied so that it is more difficult to see, more difficult to distinguish details, and more difficult to see things in their proper places. When I look at an object it may appear to me to be in one place, then the object sort of moves and so I may reach for something only to have it not be where I think it is. At this point I cannot read and I use a sub-band radio to listen to daily newspapers being read and use books on tape.

In addition to the atrophy that has occurred in the posterior part of my brain, there has also been some atrophy in the part of the brain where words are located or that helps me say words correctly. Therefore I sometimes have difficulty "finding" words or pronouncing the word I want in a standard way. Usually people around me can understand what I mean or what I meant to say. I also have some difficulty with short-term memory, but that appears to be very minimal at this point.

CHOICES

Bill Lyons

This piece originally appeared in *The Cider Press Review*

Now that a doctor has predicted
I may not live much longer,
I'll do things enjoyed, intended—
see the St. Louis Cardinals,

photograph Great Blue Herons,
read till I'm someone else,
fish for walleye in the Boundary
Waters of northern Minnesota.

Or, better, I'll sit people down,
look them in the eye, ask questions,
listen to their stories, nod, smile,
laugh, say tell it again and what

about that story you told yesterday
and last week and remember that one
you said was a favorite—when you
took the last piece of pie and your

sister chased you round and round
the house till you turned and threw
the pie in her face? Did she repay you?
Does she remember that story?

And what about the time your dad
killed the ringworm-cat with a hammer?
And when you leaned back against an open
flame on the stove, your shirt caught fire

and your mom put out the flames
with her bare hands? And vacations?
you said you slept on air mattresses
in parking lots—and traveled all over

the United States? And you and your brother
wrestled on the twin beds and how winning
meant pushing the other guy between the beds?
What other love stories do you have?

Mental Acuity Tests

Bill Lyons

This poem originally appeared in *360 Degrees*.

neurologists ask who is president?
day and date? spell world backwards
study for the test? d-l-r-o-w d-l-r-o-w
studying makes the test inaccurate

but so what meds only moderate symptoms
people with failing memories (I've heard)
remember language longer if it comes within a song
I can imagine a neurologist asking me

to sing a song I know by heart
"My home town is a one horse town
but it's good enough for me, *doop* doop, *doop* doop, *doop*-pa-doop, *doop* . . ."

and the neurologist thinks with a smile, "Ah ha!
can't remember words even in a favorite song."
and I'll get to say, "Those *are* the words
my family always sings."

Skis

Pat Healy

A pair of snow skis hanging on a hook in the garage next to the ice skates. A reminder of the reality of a diagnosis five years ago. The snow skis had not moved for five years. A fairly active woman had left them hanging in hopes of skiing again someday. Nearby the skis were other recreational touring sporting goods. A pair of roller blades, a tennis racket, a road bike, and beside them were old running shoes with soles that were slightly worn.

How did these objects find themselves together in the garage? Why were they left there? Who used these recreational items last? What had been stopping them from being moved off the garage wall and storage shelves? The journey these items had revealed was that of an active younger woman. She was reaching her prime time of forty-five years, had actually participated in one tri-athalon. Yes, she swam, biked, and ran in a mini-tri-athalon. Why would she stop being active? What could have interfered?

It was five years ago that she discovered Parkinson's disease would become a part of her life. Looking back she contemplated how many changes her life had experienced and wondered how many more times it would change.

Looking back she recalled skiing in the beautiful Colorado mountains. What caused her downhill skiing to be harder than the previous trip? Why was her left side slow to react? Why was she falling more this time? There was fresh powder snow. Could that be the reason?

After this snow experience, she began to question why she had the sense of weakness and the tremors. After a long search for the answer, three MRIs and a neurologist was seen in her home town. MS was the first suspicion but it was eventually ruled out. Finally, a practicing internist diagnosed her with fibermialgia.

After Diagnosis—What?

Pat Healy

After a long search for an answer and many tests, the feared disease of MS was negative. But searching for answers was not new to her. Fifteen years ago she had begun feeling fatigue and pain which led her to an internist who diagnosed her with fibromyalgia. For the first three years she fought the diagnosis. She did not like being labeled, especially if this was such a new disease and it would become part of a medical record. She did learn a lot by reading about it. She definitely fit the symptoms, aching joints and chronic pain. What is fibromyalgia? Why would the doctor believe she had this new disease? What did it mean—how would it affect her? The doctor offered a support group. She attended a meeting. It horrified her, as many at the meeting were more advanced, totally disabled or badly crippled. She fought hard, not to fit the mold of fibromyalgia patients.

She lived in denial and experienced anger about the disease. She felt loss and had little hope. She tried to convince herself that someday all of this would stop and she would be her old self again.

The tremors began to be more frequent and pronounced. She felt internal and external tremors. It was miserable for her. But worse still was the feeling that she was losing control of her body and its fight for balance in her life. Her posture and body weight were changing and she didn't know why. She began to have other health problems. Female problems led to a hysterectomy. She could not understand why and how all these health issues suddenly surfaced. Was it coincidental or were they all related? When would she find the answer? Did she really want to know the answer?

To make matters worse, she began to become frustrated with her art teaching position. The job that was once exciting and rewarding because of the diversity now seemed to be out of control. What was once her passion, had now become a job. Her love of art and love of people gave her great interactions for twenty years. But these last three years had become increasingly challenging and frustrating. What was going on? The struggle to balance her life with her health caused her a great amount of pain: physical and emotional. What had become of the quality of life and well being?

Struggling at her job, she continued to teach. She began to hate her job; she was overwhelmed and fatigued. The doctor visits and tests continued for several years until finally the neurologist observed classic Parkinson's symptoms, tremors on the side of her body. The left side was slow and the tremors were on the left side as well. The left arm did not swing at her side as she walked which gave the doctor a pretty good idea that it was in fact Parkinson's. However, the doctor would need to try Parkinson's medications to be assured the diagnosis was correct.

The doctor treated the physical symptoms but what was the difficulty at work? Why were the classroom and preparations so overwhelming? The physical symptoms were being controlled by medicine. But this didn't explain the confusion and the overwhelming emotions. Side effects from the medicine caused difficulties. It was a challenge to determine which of the medicines was causing the physical reactions. It was during this time that the doctor recommended her to go on disability from her teaching position.

After nine months of adjusting and experimenting with her medications it was obvious that her Parkinson's had affected some of her cognitive skills as the doctor had proven by skill testing. The tests showed that multi-tasking was difficult if not impossible. This was devastating to her and yet she had no choice but to step down from teaching. It was both sad and yet a relief; it felt humiliating, yet she tried to leave with a good reputation. She wrote a letter of resignation and it was received for consideration. The letter she wrote also had a copy of the doctor's recommendation letter. It was a short time before the administration and school board acted on the request. She was officially retired from teaching. The most difficult task of her teaching career was walking away from the students and staff she loved. She decided to leave the position with her head held high, on angels' wings, which gave her the strength to walk away from the job before the school year ended.

Currently she is creating her own art and enjoying retirement. Still faced with the multiple task challenges. Grateful for the disease to be progressing slowly and hopeful that science will stay ahead of the progression. She is still driven by spiritual strength and encouraged by affirmations on a regular basis. She has a desire to help others and to be an active part of the community. She uses her creativity to support fundraisers in the community, as well as to support the fine arts. Her age is currently fifty. She figures there is a fifty/fifty chance on her progression of the disease. She is younger than most who have Parkinson's which will allow her to fight for better and better health. The mind is a powerful tool that she plans to use. She believes in the phrase: "use it or lose it." You simply can't give up. Hope and faith will light her way.

I Have Such a Wonderful Life

Earl Rose

"I have such a wonderful life!" said Rachel, our 14-year-old granddaughter. This is an adolescent who is facing many challenges. She is a high school freshman who weighs fifty pounds and is fifty inches tall. She had surgery and is undergoing treatment for a tumor at the base of her brain in proximity to the pituitary gland—a craniopharyngioma—the cause of her small size.

As I look back to my learning of my diagnosis of Parkinson's Disease, I had some self-pity. It was diagnosed delayed, and as I mentally reviewed the occasion it was a diagnosis made with a bit of reluctance by my physicians. I, however, was relieved to know the diagnosis for then I could make some plans. This diagnosis was made when I was seventy-nine years old. What of my tremors, imbalance, slowness, and debility as compared to my granddaughter.

My first question following the diagnosis was the natural history and progression of this degenerative disorder. To my surprise I find survival periods variable; some have an apparent arrested condition with life for years and death customarily from an intervening condition such as Pope John Paul experienced. Parkinson's does not appear to have a predictable timetable or schedule. Is this more ominous than the slowly evolving disease? Or a rapidly progressive condition?

A feeling of being of worth is important to me, so I must search for ways and activities that will enhance my sense of worth. There is one activity that I consider of primacy—that is making choices to be my better self and to savor the many pleasures available. I too can have a wonderful life.

Parkinson's Disease:
There is Life Before Death

Earl Rose

I am pleased to participate in this group of persons with Parkinson's disease in which we document "our journey" and share our thoughts of the journey. This is a way of coming to grips with my present reality and to plan, explore and acknowledge the future. This should be every bit as exciting as our pasts, though the downside of this present equation is the more compelling.

My preliminary reaction to the diagnosis of Parkinson's mirrored that of Mark Twain who, on the death of his invalid daughter, observed bitterly that "She was now set free from the swindle of this life." With a moment's reflection, I cannot look on my diagnosis and symptoms with bitterness, rancor or anger, and certainly I have not been swindled by a lifetime of experiences and opportunities. My wife and I look to the future with some apprehension, but we have given up fear, and know that the chronicles of death are written of in many contexts, some of which we do not find credible. We live confronted by the caveat that death is the condition of our birth.

> The abundant life is defined by its quality and not its quantity. In that spirit, we seek to live each day as fully and as joyfully as we can in spite of the uncertainties we face. May we all remain people of hope rather than despair.

Rodney Sawatsky, President of Messiah College, Grantham, PA. He died Nov. 27, 2004 at age 60 from complications of a brain tumor.

To host a slowly progressive condition such as Parkinson's disease demands a bit of getting used to it. Arriving at the conclusion that there is life before death was a preliminary step for me and if I am to treat Parkinson's disease as a condition with which I must become intimate and familiar. It is now a constant companion who makes demands, e.g.; a cane for balance. Failure to include my "third leg" can bring a sudden reminder such as a stum-

40

ble or a fall. This "staff of balance" is accompanied by a limp and decisions such as which hand to use to hold the cane. Tremors quietly invade my frame and bring loss of my previously prized dexterity—tremors that masquerade as pure clumsiness.

I know that Parkinson's disease shall be neither my mistress nor my master. Perhaps time will despoil this bravado and I shall indeed be brought low.

Walking Sticks/Canes

Earl and Marilyn Rose

"Walking stick or cane," are names used interchangeably to describe one of the oldest tools used by mankind to lighten the burden, provide purchase and economize energy expenditure. In addition to support for the body, canes/walking sticks are among the earliest utilitarian tools. Man first pushed himself upright to the walking position, and permitted transportation and manipulation of untold objects used in daily living. Certainly on par with the inclined plane. It was a useful evolutionary tool, and some have claimed this was an early manifestation of creationism (at least there was a superior mind involved). The walking stick is also rapidly adaptable into a weapon of defense. One can fend off dogs or other domesticated animals, muggers, or even an Absalom (II Samuel 18:19) or other low hanging branch.

The "cane" is a type of walking stick with the shaft shorter than the "typical" walking stick, and is customarily thicker and tapered. The appropriate length can be determined by holding the cane upside down with the ferule at a point where the hip joint projects. It is frequently an accoutrement of evening clothes. It may be decorated with precious jewels and handsome carvings or inlays of ivory, metal of mother-of-pearl.

A ferule of brass usually is fitted over the distal end of the shaft to prevent rapid wear and to provide a good hold. When adopted by rulers it may be called a scepter.

The typical "walking stick" customarily is 36 inches long and ¾ inches thick; however this is variable. It is not tapered. If it is four feet or taller it greatly augments balance by acting as a third leg. They may have a curved ledge on the handle to rest the thumb. Walking sticks, thought, perhaps more utilitarian, may be intricately carved and decorated. The finish is usually linseed oil with a final coat of spar varnish. Margaret Mead, a famous anthropologist, always carried a walking stick, even when giving public lectures.

The handles of both canes and walking sticks are variable and may be very decorative. They may be part of the stick (self handle) or may be attached with metal, antlers, wood or any material that provides a comfortable handhold.

There are various types of walking sticks such as the hiking staff, and the shepherd's crook that is at least 28 inches long. The shepherd's crook has a crook as a handle—it may be a neck crook or a leg cleek (a large hook which may be used to grasp—and a #1 golf club is also called a cleek). There are also wading poles; tipple sticks that contain a flask and shooting sticks, i.e., a cane pointed at one end with a folding seat at the other, typically used by spectators at outdoor sporting events.

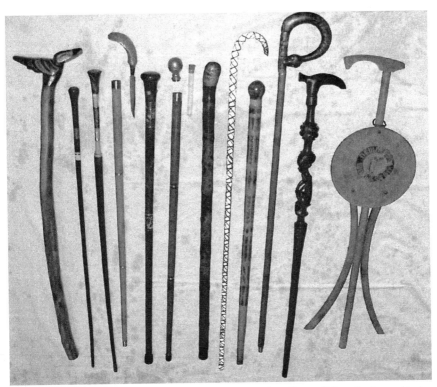

Examples from our collection. Left to right: Raven handle—self handle from Alaska, Leather wrapped "whip" from Ft. Madison, Brass and mother-of-pearl "umbrella" handle, Brass cobra with knife insert, Cloisonné and carving from China, Ball-shaped brass handle with flask, Black lacquered and carved from China, Glass cane from England, Oak with decorative inlay of other woods, Snake striking self from Pakistan, Carved ebony figure with mother-of-pearl inlay from Mozambique, and Shooting Stick.

The Once and Future Caregiver

Caryl Lyons

I've been a caregiver before, so I have some idea of what it's all about. My husband, Bill Lyons, was diagnosed with leukemia in 2000, he had stem cell infusion, spent 100 days in the hospital, and came home with intravenous nutrition and three kinds of intravenous medications to take. He was so weak he couldn't get up by himself. We slept in our family room since he couldn't climb steps. I had to time the intravenous nutrition and medications exactly so that they fit in between when I arrived home from work and when I had to leave again the next morning. Of course, I had to do everything that needed to be done around the house, to answer the many phone and e-mail messages that came on a daily basis to check on Bill's current status, to cook and wash clothes and do all the routine tasks that we had shared. I had to get up with him in the night, many times each night.

But I learned what was vital and what was just "nice" to do. I learned to go right back to sleep after getting up. I learned to concentrate at work even better than I ever had, in order, perhaps, to give myself a bit of a break from caregiving. I learned to accept help gratefully from friends and colleagues. I learned to pace myself and take time to enjoy whatever we could enjoy together, whether it was watching a basketball game on television or listening to music or reading poetry aloud. One day I came home from work to find that I had received a Caregiver Award, a plaque from "The Council of Grateful and Impressed Spouses" signed by my "grateful and impressed spouse," carefully printed out on our computer and framed, "For demonstrated affection, love, caring, patience, and extra time and energy in the face of additional work"—October 13, 2000.

Then Bill recovered from the leukemia and most of the side affects of the chemotherapy. Having lost ninety-five pounds, he gained back fifty to end up

44

at 180 pounds, about what he was when we first got married. His mouth sores healed, the lesions on his skin recovered, he grew new fingernails and toenails to replace the ones he had lost. He gained enough strength to again take walks and ride the exercise bicycle. He had never lost his sense of humor or his appreciation of life even at its worst. He was able to take charge of his own medications again, to drive again, to go to movies after his blood counts got good enough that he no longer had to be so careful around groups of people and their illnesses. He could even do a few errands, and I saw my life as a caregiver disappearing.

Then, a few months later, he lost a significant amount of his vision. Still no one knows what caused part of his optic nerve to atrophy, though it may well have been another result of the chemotherapy. Driving for him was still legal, but when he realized that his blind spots were obscuring everything from a child on a bike to a semi, when it was in the right, or rather the wrong, place in his field of vision, he voluntarily quit driving, and I was back to being a caregiver in that regard, even sooner than I would have been had he waited on the progression of Parkinson's symptoms. He had to stay home more now, but while I was functioning as the caregiver in some ways, he was functioning as mine, while I continued to work. I try to do little things that I can do quickly, the things that take much longer for a person with Parkinson's disease; buttoning shirts, writing addresses on envelopes.

It's four years later, and the Parkinson's has, of course, progressed some. But I still feel as though I'm in my honeymoon period as a caregiver. Most of what I can do for Bill is in the realm of ways I can spend time with him. The one hundred days he spent in the hospital with leukemia gave me a deep appreciation of his presence. I continue to do all the driving, though once Bill gets to Iowa City or Coralville from North Liberty, he has become expert on the bus systems, including Cambus, which goes to University Hospitals. I do most of the errands, but sometimes he feels like going, too. He handles all his own transportation arrangements. We enjoy doing many things together.

I participated in a survey of caregivers of those with Parkinson's disease a year or so ago and recently received a copy of the results. It discusses many of the problems faced by both persons with PD and their caregivers, mostly things you would expect—the ways people learn to compromise, to adapt their lifestyles and their future plans to their new realities. The ways that Parkinson's symptoms get confused with symptoms of aging. The ways that caregivers and those who have Parkinson's struggle with balancing the need for help with the need for independence. But the most interesting thing to me were the lines from the end of the "caregiver" section. "Importantly, a majority of caregivers took pride in their ability to provide assistance to their spouse. They enjoyed their 'one-on-one time' and were pleased that they were able to support their partner even under stressful conditions."

The once and future caregiver. T. H. White's book about King Arthur is called *The Once and Future King*. Once I was a caregiver. Now I am a bit of a caregiver. In the future, I expect to be more of a caregiver. Recently, I read an excerpt from Joan Didion's new book *The Year of Magical Thinking*, which is about the death of her husband, suddenly and without warning, as they were sitting down to dinner. He had a massive coronary and was gone before he could say anything. I'm grateful for the more than five years I've had with Bill since we thought he might not survive his stem cell infusion. Caregiving may have its ups and downs, but I hope to be a caregiver for a very long time yet.

To Caryl—Caregiver

Bill Lyons

Your being a caregiver when I had leukemia
helped me to live. Now you have taken on
the caregiver role again, this time for a

Parkinson's patient. I have a special interest
in your willingness to serve in this role, your
generosity of spirit, since I am the patient again.

Is this what the minister meant when he said
"for better or for worse, till death do us part"?
I know I'm still in the "honeymoon" period

in terms of Parkinson's symptoms: tremor,
fatigue, cramped handwriting, slow movement
including slow eating, and unsteady balance.

But as I anticipate additional symptoms
over the years, my courage is strengthened
by your presence, your humor, your love.

Thanks for taking on the caregiver role, Caryl.
May your courage, and your energy,
be strengthened by my love for you.

Just Say "Thanks": A Prose Poem

Bob McCown

Fourteen years after I was diagnosed with Parkinson's disease, I continue to carry on despite some hardships. More than just existing, I am actually doing quite satisfactorily. The reason for my well being is not answered by an ontological discussion, but by more down to earth explanations. Because of my diminished energy, I rely on my wife to be my caregiver. In addition, friends, acquaintances, and even strangers give strength and hope to me and alleviate my discomforts. For all of these acts, I am appreciative. Showing gratitude has not come easy to me. I have not said "Thank you" often enough. So, while I still have joy in being alive, I must continue to grow as a person by being more thankful. I have so many things to be grateful for: a loving wife, children, grandchildren, an extended family, and friends; a roof over my head, clothes on my back, and nourishment in my stomach; long walks and good books; and a beautiful world for my eyes to see. I cannot say "Thank you" often enough. So, the next time you see me, count the number of times I say "Thanks!"

Part II

Showing Respect through Creative Interchange[1]

Bill Lyons

This I believe:

- every person is worthy of respect
- respect for another person grows out of knowledge of that person's ideas and culture
- interaction with others must accompany knowledge about them
- and that a workable kind of interaction was described by Henry Nelson Wieman, Unitarian philosopher and theologian

Wieman said that through a process he called "creative interchange," people can learn from each other and about each other, accepting the good and integrating it into their own personality, and rejecting the bad.

How to distinguish good from bad, according to Wieman? Bad things, if carried out infinitely, tend to destroy themselves. Examples: suspicion, hatred, war, preemptive strikes. Good things, if carried out infinitely, continue to exist. Examples: peace, love, helping others, perhaps the act of writing, especially in its role as a clarifier of the writer's ideas. James Van Allen said, "I am never as clear about a matter as when I have just finished writing about it . . . The writing process itself is a powerful technique for consolidating and advancing one's own understanding" (*Iowa City Press-Citizen*, April 28, 1979). Thus, writing may promote the process of creative interchange by helping the writer clarify if and what transformation is taking place.

While teaching at the University of Chicago, Wieman dedicated himself to what he understood to be the central problem in religious inquiry: he wanted to seek a better understanding of the nature of whatever it is in human life and experience that transforms us in ways that we cannot transform ourselves.

Wieman came to believe that we are transformed by this process called "Creative Interchange," or "God." If the word God is used, I prefer it to mean the power which allows people to experience the process of creative interchange. If my labeling myself an atheist, Christian, Muslim, or something else interferes with someone talking with me, I do not argue about "my label." Rather, I downplay whatever label others associate with me, in favor of engaging in creative interchange and learning as much as I can about other people and cultures. So, I do not avoid using the word God. Rather, I use it in the context of discussing the power humans have been given to learn from each other.

In *The Source of Human Good*, Wieman defines "creative interchange" as a single "event," with four stages:

1. Emerging awareness of another's perspective.
2. Integrating this new awareness with existing knowledge.
3. There is expansion and enrichment of what is known and valued because of this new awareness.
4. Finally, there is a widening and deepening of mutual understanding.

I'd like to note these four stages of creative interchange one more time.

In the first stage, Wieman describes an "emerging awareness"—listening to people and becoming aware of a different perspective, as they share significant stories about who they are.

The second stage is integrating this emerging awareness, this new perspective, into our existing understandings. You come to value and understand this other perspective for what it is, on its own terms.

The third stage involves expanding and enriching one's understanding of the world. Wieman comments, "If this new understanding/meaning has been creatively integrated, the individual sees what he could not see before; she feels what she could not feel before." As a result, new structures of interrelatedness are formed between individuals and groups.

The fourth stage is the widening and deepening of the community, which grows because your sense of self grows as you understand more and more of the community.

When I use the word "community," I wish to promote a sense of INclusiveness rather than EXclusiveness. As I struggle with this idea, the concept of "shared values" somehow does not seem inclusive enough to promote peace and harmony in a broader community, perhaps even a world community. Unless, unless, people could agree that the process of creative interchange might smooth the way.

So, what might a favorable condition be, for nurturing creative interchange? Any situation that promotes open discussion, any group that helps us understand each other. How can we as individuals promote a desire to interact in the spirit of creative interchange? Here are two examples you might not think of.

A woman told me the most remarkable story about her son when he was in Stu Sheeley's eighth-grade class. The son said, "Mom, don't ever tell Mr. Sheeley that I'm not as smart as he thinks I am." Mr. Sheeley may have been thinking that some people need to succeed before they can learn.

Is this an example of creative interchange? I'm not sure. But it ties in with an idea promoted by the Iowa Writing Project (for teachers), that writers may benefit from having their writing examined, first, in terms of what can be honestly praised, before the writing is broadly critiqued. In both instances, something positive has been initiated that may help people engage in creative interchange. The University of Iowa's Writers' Workshop favors a less structured approach.

Does the Golden Rule promote creative interchange? Only if the other person really does wish to be done unto as you would have others do unto you. If I am trying to learn about another person, I might be better guided if I follow the "Silver Rule"—Do unto others as they would have you do unto them.

I hope you will share some of your creative interchange strategies with me and with whoever else you can get to listen, oops, I mean whoever you can get to talk with you.

NOTE

1. This paper was presented originally as a talk, one in a series of "This I Believe" statements.

Trust or Distrust

Otto Bauer

When confronted with the concepts "trust' or "distrust," treating them as bipolar options is very tempting. Unfortunately, we engage in so much "either-or" thinking that we begin to convince ourselves that the world around us can be described, for example, as good or bad, right or wrong, rich or poor, beautiful or ugly, or smart or dumb. When we stop for a moment and reflect upon these options, we quickly realize that concepts like "trust or distrust," like those other oppositions, exist on a continuum, where it is much more helpful, meaningful, and accurate to ask, how much trust or distrust you have in a given person, organization, or situation, rather than trying to push the judgment to one of its polar extremes. In real life, these concepts usually exist as a blending of ideas and feelings. It makes much more sense to ask, to what extent are these persons, places, things, or actions good or bad, right or wrong, or rich or poor?

Similarly, we have a tendency to look for the meaning of a given concept or word. In real life, we know that words have many meanings and often the intended meanings are only clear from the context in which they are used. The word "fast," for example, can have exactly the opposite meanings. Describing an airplane as "fast" could comment on its ability to go quickly from one place to another or, on the other hand, could comment on its being tied down and going nowhere. And although it sounds the same, you are describing two quite different notions when your intention is to either "raise" or "raze" a building.

So, why search for single meanings for trust and distrust? Realize that these are very complex concepts that can have many meanings to many persons in many contexts or situations. As indicated in the previous essay, trust in interpersonal relations can be defined as the expectation that a person's comments and actions will exemplify competence, integrity, and good will. And although its bipolar counterpart, distrust, can be described as the expectation that a person's comments or actions will exemplify incompetence, deceit, and bad intentions, we know that any given comment or action can be located somewhere along the continuum between the two extremes of total trust or total distrust. Placing "win" on one end of a continuum and "lose" on the other can leave room for other kinds of victories and losses, such as ties, blowouts, mistakes, scandals, forfeits, fraud, etc. So-called "bottom-line thinkers," who argue that winning at any cost is justified, are loathe to admit these other possibilities, but they can be much more descriptive of what happened than the simple "win" or "lose."

Putting people together, or adding-up interpersonal relationships, results in the building of a society or a culture. Some of the organizations that develop are industries, businesses, political parties, governments, religions, terrorist cells, etc. The trusting expectation that a person's comments and actions will exemplify competence, integrity, and good-will also applies to organizations in our society: societal trust. Like individuals, organizations in a society may also exhibit untrustworthy behavior, exemplified by incompetence, deceit, and bad intentions. It is true, however, that along the path between society trust and distrust are the actions of one or more human beings; organizations do not exist in a vacuum, void of human participation.

The second major definition of trust identified is the expectation, or trust, we have in the technical competence of given individuals (interpersonal trust) and of corporations or businesses (societal trust) to create products and provide services that are effective and efficient, with minimum harm to persons and the environment. Distrust results when persons are unable to rely upon the expected performance of these products or services, such as the number of Bridgestone tires that failed on Ford Explorers at high speeds in high temperature locales. Every time we ride an elevator or any other mode of transportation, we place our trust in the technical competence of the people who design, build, operate, and service these products.

The third definition of trust identified is the expectation that persons and organizations will accept their fiduciary responsibility to follow the accepted norms of a given culture or society. The trustee of a trust fund has the responsibility to manage that fund in the best interests of the client, i.e., to select securities wisely in order to assure the maximum return on investment, consistent with the client's objectives. Initiating or approving expenditures from the trust fund that involve a conflict of interest by the trustee, such as making investments in businesses or companies in which the trustee has a financial interest, approving unreasonable fees submitted by executors of an estate, or charging unreasonable fees for managing the fund are examples of violating a fiduciary responsibility.

Distrust results when persons do not accept the fiduciary responsibility to follow the cultural norms needed to develop the economic, political, and social structures of a given society. Non-acceptance can lead to the problems of how to catch persons who try to drive away from a gasoline station without paying for the gas or who try to leave a restaurant without paying the bill.

On the international level, an expectation exists that nations will follow international law, pursuing peaceful relations with their neighbors, and treating their own people in humanitarian ways. Examples of distrust abound, including open warfare as well as various restrictions in trade.

From a review of the literature, there is little doubt that trust has a very powerful, positive impact on a society and that distrust has a very powerful negative impact. While our objective should be to develop as much trust as possible, we have to face the reality that untrustworthy behavior will continue to occur. If trust were the dominant practice in a society, we could, for example, expect few if any major acts of war or terrorism. But the reality of living in our world is the likelihood that some individuals and groups have developed sufficient hatred of the U.S. and Americans that their distrust has resulted in major acts of terrorism.

While we may choose to travel the more honorable path of fostering trust, we still need to recognize that we are likely to be faced with many acts that represent distrust, and we must prepare ourselves to live as best we can with the constant threat of violence. An old saying comes to mind: "Hope for the best, but expect the worst."

As indicated above in the discussion of the first definition of trust, Aristotle identified the ethical appeal of a person (ethos) as the most powerful tool of persuasion. People are swayed mightily by the assumed credibility of a person. Placed in a somewhat later context, Bryce Harlow, formerly an adviser to President Nixon, challenged George Schultz to remember one thing: "Trust is the coin of the realm; trust is the coin of the realm." Sociologist Neva R. Goodwin reached for a different analogy in her comment that "Trust is as essential in the context of business as it is in other human relations; it is the grease that keeps the wheels turning. Responsibility, however, is an important part of what makes trust possible."

Being responsible for one's comments and actions is a particularly strong way of fostering trust. But living in a society where many have come to distrust first and to trust later, only after it is earned, requires that a person also be willing to be held accountable for his or her actions by opening necessary records, disclosing important information, and not trying to ensure total privacy.

It is important to note that fostering trust and at the same time learning to live with distrust are not necessarily opposite ends of a continuum. Most persons will find themselves trying to live in a positive manner with all of the elements identified by these three definitions of trust. Pursuing trusting relationships can enhance labor-management negotiations, improve courtroom proceedings, and promote agreement among political adversaries. All of these actions can assist greatly in reducing distrusting relationships. But this effort is in search of an ideal of perfect trustworthiness, which simply cannot be reached. Try as we may, human perfection will not occur.

Beatitude

by Earl Rose

I respected Mr. Lewis, respected him a great deal for he had "paid his dues" and turned the other cheek many times over. His professional goals were of necessity modest as he was a black man in the South in the 1960s. My acquaintance with him rested on his role as an accomplished toxicologist at Parkland Hospital where we were colleagues in the Forensic Sciences. His aspirations were truncated by bigotry, geography, the times and politics of the South. Mr. Lewis was competent, courteous, remote and quietly dignified. His hair was graying and thinning; his eyes were bright and penetrating; and he was portly which gave him the appearance of strength not of obesity.

The city had many problems, the most pressing at that time was school integration. The newspaper reported a vocal, aggressive and potentially threatening gathering in the black section of the city. This gathering consisted of the black community members and a few white city leaders. In the newspaper account of the meeting was a picture of Mr. Lewis in the front row. Their demands were for fairness for the black school children. He was not only articulate but had the strength of will and purpose to speak out publicly—such courage.

The next day I went to visit him at the Hospital Laboratory and asked him "How is it that you, a committed leader in the Black community, have the strength and courage to press your will for what is obviously right but potentially self-destructive if pushed? Why do you do this when there is nothing in it for you?" I remember he stood next to the lab bench and after much thought shared an answer of wisdom—"If you don't do nothing, you can't be right." This has become a yardstick against which I measure my actions.

Writing From Prison

David Belgum

Writing from prison is nothing new. While in prison Saint Paul wrote a pastoral counseling letter to Philemon advising him how to treat his slave, Onesimus. Dietrich Bonhoeffer, the anti-Nazi theologian, wrote *Letters and Papers From Prison.* From Birmingham jail, Martin Luther King, Jr. wrote advocating non-violent resistance to racial injustice. Some have written autobiographical accounts of a conversion experience like Charles Colson (*Born Again* Chosen Books, Inc. 1976).

An active group supporting writing that is known by the acronym, PEN (Poets Playwrights, Essayists, Editors and Novelists), published *Doing Time, 25 Years of Prison Writing* (Edited by Bell Gale Chevigny, 1999). Also an amazingly ambitious program was conducted in San Quentin Prison. For four years Judith Tannenbaum conducted a weekly class in poetry for ten inmates, some under life sentence. The climax came about when the play, *Waiting for Godot*, was performed by the inmates. Several performances were attended by an audience of 1,400 including inmates, the public, and journalists reporting on the entire project.

The Borderline Between Interpretation and Confidentiality

David Belgum

Oxford University Press has done a good job in this regard, i.e., *The Border-line Between Interpretation and Confidentiality. With Injured Brains of Medical Minds*. The author of one chapter describing an officer leaving the Navy to return to general practice, simply signs the article as "Anonymous." He wants to share his story but at the same time does not want to undermine his professional reputation. Weird behavior can be left to the circus or comedy stage.

Another author, who has a nurses aide status, stresses all the things that can go wrong. *Views from Within* is the sub-title of the Oxford book. It is not the case that the brain tissue is different in physicians from brain tissue in the brains of the laity. It is a matter of perspective. A brain surgeon, who has many procedures, is aware of the complications that are present in some cases but not in others. Let us explore how to give the actors individuality and believability, yet abide by the guiding rules in fiction that provide good individual character without violating confidentiality. Go ahead, try it!

Loose Canoe

Bill Lyons

The beginnings of the Meramec River in eastern Missouri offer pleasant but lively canoeing opportunities. The channel is often narrow and swift, and capsizing is not uncommon. But the river is popular, and help is usually nearby, whether needed or not.

Early in one of our trips, we rounded a bend and found a hundred-foot long sandbar with maybe a dozen couples eating lunch, fishing or just enjoying a beautiful September day. The channel cut sharply to the right through small rapids, then continued around the sandbar to form a semicircle. In the rough water, we lost control of our canoe and capsized. The river was over our heads, but after some serious floundering, we were able to grab hold of the gunnels. Soon our feet touched the river bottom, and we walked the canoe to shore. We were safe, but an ice chest and pack full of our picnic supplies were bobbing down the river around the bend.

Before we could think about trying to retrieve our floating gear, teenage voices rang out, "Don't worry. We'll get your stuff for you!" Two high school boys were in fact heading quickly for the river, with their canoe, intending to rescue our ice chest and pack.

They waded into the swift water, pushing their empty canoe, thinking to grab our gear and throw it into their canoe, but the current wrestled their canoe away from them and sent it heading rapidly around the sandbar. "Loose canoe" a nearby fisherman yelled at the top of his lungs.

Every male on that sandbar responded to the call. It was as though Michael Jordan was leading a fast break and everyone else was racing down court to fill an outside lane in the hopes of making the lay-up at the other end. "Sprint" a voice in each head urged. And sprint they did, young men running hard across that sandbar to where the river completed its semicircle and straightened out. That looked like the point where they could intercept the canoe.

But there was little time, and as feet pounded the sand and voices continued to cry—"Loose canoe"—each runner realized he would have to dive into the river to grab the canoe before it hit the deep fast channel at the end of the sandbar. "Dive" cried the voices. "Grab it." And we did. Yes, I was there, too. Ten of us, five on each side, grasped the canoe by the gunnels. We were in control, or were we? Too late we realized that we could not touch the river bottom, the current had picked up, and we were all being swept downstream.

We clung to the gunnels, our bodies hanging in the water, our eyes staring across the top of the canoe at strangers, as the river swept us out of sight of the cheering spectators left behind on the sandbar. Guys who try to be macho but fail are not likely to see the humor in defeat, and so our few laughs were drown out by profanities. But all of us, strangers to each other, felt a sense of oneness, of unity of purpose, as we tried to "beat the river." We were swept down river eighty yards before we could guide the canoe to the next sandbar. Now the question was, how to rejoin the people left behind. The bank beyond this new sandbar was steep and heavily wooded and the current was fast. Two young guys tried to paddle up river but capsized. Three of us then got into the canoe and tried pulling ourselves through the branches overhanging the water along the shore. Then we pushed and shoved the canoe up the fifteen-foot bank to portage through the woods.

But by then the left-behind canoeists had gotten the remaining boats into the water and were floating down to pick us up. "Sorry to break up the party," I said to the assembled group.

"Hey, that's all right," said one of the boys who had earlier pushed the empty canoe into the current and started the big chase down the river. "I never knew what 'loose canoe' meant before. I learned a couple of things today." We laughed and then headed back down the Meramec, knowing that if we needed help it was all too ready.

Building a Canoe of My Own

David Good

I have always had an interest in water. When I was 11 years old I saw my first canoe and learned that it was built by the owner. The owner was a member of a scout troop that had been building canoes for the last fifteen years.

Having seen this owner-built canoe I wanted to learn how to build a canoe for myself. I was in luck as I was in line to become a member of the canoe building Scout Troop 4 in Lincoln, Nebraska, where I lived.

The person who had the ultimate knowledge of canoe building was a man who worked for the Department of Education for the state of Nebraska. His name was Mr. Rosine. He was one of the scout leaders. Mr. Rosine allowed his basement to be used as the workshop for building canoes. He lived about ten blocks away from the house where I lived and close to the campus of Nebraska Wesleyan University. At the same time I was building my canoe, four or five of my friends and their dads were also building canoes in Mr. Rosine's basement. We worked individually, but as a group.

I saved up my money to be able to pay for the materials that had to be purchased to build the canoe. The needed structural materials were white pine and second growth ash. The white pine was purchased from the local lumber yard. It was cut into thin slats long enough for the length of the canoe. We found the second growth ash on land by the Platte River. We cut down the trees and took them to a mill where we planed them and cut them up. The second growth ash was used for the middle of the canoe frame.

We started construction. We created the frame of the canoe by nailing the pine and the ash together. The ash was used to build the frame because it was more pliable and stronger. The pine was used to fill in the structure of the canoe. Once the structure was completed the slats were treated with linseed oil. It had to dry.

Then we had to cover the canoe with canvas by tacking it to the slats. We shrunk the canvas, to get it taut, by getting the canvas wet. Once the covering was taut, the next step was to paint the exterior. We used airplane paint. I originally chose orange paint. I just always liked the color orange. I think the actual name of the color was arunka orange. Sometime later in my life I repainted the canoe so now it is red.

At the same time we made the canoes we also made our paddles using a band saw. They were made of pine. They had to be shaped and sanded. It took many hours.

Once the canoes were built we took them to the Platte River, christened them and put them to the test. We put in at Lincoln Beach. There were two people per canoe. My dad was the second person in my canoe because he had helped me with the process.

We paddled down the river. We stayed overnight on the banks of the Platte River. The next day we continued to Plattesmith on the Missouri River where we took the canoes out.

I believe Mr. Rosine put the number on each canoe when it was finished, signifying how many canoes he had guided to completion. I think my canoe was number 114. He continued to help scouts like me build canoes long after he helped me.

In addition to canoeing on the Platte and Missouri Rivers, several times I took my canoe to the Boundary Waters and into Canada on scouting trips. My dad and other scouts were part of those trips too.

With Mr. Rosine's help we also made our own packs. We got surplus army green canvas left over from World War II. Neil Slack, a professor at Nebraska Wesleyan University, did the majority of the sewing work. I think that as a scout I helped some. We called the packs elephant packs.

I was very excited to have the opportunity to know people like Mr. Rosine and Mr. Slack who were doers. They were very organized. They'd figure out how to get materials as inexpensively as they could. For example, Mr. Slack figured out how to make the packs out of the surplus canvas.

I always wanted to be doing things so I really like that these guys were doers and would help me do exciting things.

Some of the work on the canoes demanded cooperation from everyone. We all would help stretch the canvas over the frames of the canoes. When we went on trips we would all have to work together to set up camp and do the cooking, etc. I thought it was great to work together.

I liked the adventure of it all. At that time on the Platte River, if the water was up, you had to watch for tree trunks and other obstacles. When we got to the Missouri River we had to navigate carefully to stay away from the big towboats and barges. It was kind of like being Tom Sawyer or Huck Finn.

Mr. Rosine and the other men that guided us made sure that the work we did was to their satisfaction and met high standards. In this process they were available to answer questions. They would observe our work and often times worked along side us to guide us.

I never had any doubts that my canoe would float when it was launched. Mr. Rosine and many scouts before me had been successful. There were no stories of a craft not floating.

This canoe building experience, which I connect to my fascination with water, gave me a lot of confidence. I'd had a prior water experience that had not given me confidence. When I was in second grade I had to learn to swim. I went to lessons at the high school. It came to the day of the lessons that I had to show that I could jump into the pool. I was wearing a swimsuit that was a hand-me-down from my older brother. It felt too big and I had tried to tell my mother about that fact but she would not listen.

I jumped into the pool. My suit came off. I had to get out of the pool sans suit. I was mortified. I took lessons in a coed group. When I got out my mother was laughing. She thought it was funny. I, of course, did not.

This swimming experience bashed my confidence so it was good to later have a positive canoe building experience that boosted my confidence.

Three Pieces From *Learning From the Lizard* and *Stories Told Under the Sycamore Tree*

Sam Hahn

Sam Hahn has written two books with devotional thoughts helpful to Parkinson's patients, or anyone struggling with health issues. His book *Learning from the Lizard*, deals with lessons from animals from the Bible and *Stories told under the Sycamore Tree* introduces lessons from plants found in the Bible. Two stories from the first and one from the second are reprinted on the following pages. Both are artistically illustrated by nature artist Scott Patton. These books are available at most local book stores or from amazon.com and from CSS Publishing. (Used by permission from CSS Publishing Company, 517 S. Main Street, Lima Ohio 45804)

HONEY BEE: A WILLING WORKER

The Laws of the Lord are just; they are always fair. They are more desirable than the finest gold; they are sweeter than the purest honey (Psalm 19:9–10 TEV).

Certainly the loving Creator had our best interest at heart when he planned to provide the rare delicacy of honey. The glowing term used to describe the Holy Land is, "a land of milk and honey." Honey is an excellent food course providing sugars that can be used quickly by the body. It is good and good for you!

The Bible refers to bees only four times, but honey is included sixty-two times. Honey producing bees are wonderful creatures that can be found worldwide, except in frigid polar areas. I have seen nature programs in which the people of some countries actually risk their lives to climb high cliffs in order to collect prized honey from the swarm's beehives.

The God-given intelligence of the bee is amazing. A colony normally has from 60,000 to 80,000 workers and one queen. There are a few drones (males) whose only function is to fertilize the queen once in her lifetime. Most of the workers are involved in collecting nectar from flowers. To make a pound of honey, they travel about 13,000 miles, or four times the distance across the United States. During her lifetime, the worker collects only one tenth of a pound of honey.

Not only do the bees provide honey, but most of our fruits and many other crops could not produce if the bee did not carry pollen from plant to plant in the collecting process.

When a worker returns to the nest after finding a potential source of nectar, it does a sort of dance before the other bees that indicates the direction in relation to the sun that the flowers can be found. Their flight pattern is amazing. They can fly forward, side-ways, backward, and can hover in one place. Once they have a load of pollen and nectar, they make a "bee line"—a very direct path back to the hive.

Interesting facts about the honey bee include: the beeswax produced from their combs is amazingly durable. Each individual part is formed with a perfect hexagon for development of the young or for honey storage. The best candles available are made from beeswax. As well as being marvelous and delicious, honey is claimed to have healing powers. It is such a pure substance that honey, still preserved, has been found in Egyptian tombs over 2,000 years old. The worker bee is willing to give up its life for the sake of the hive. Once the worker stings it loses its life. The queen can sting many times and the drone doesn't even have a stinger.

Bees have an amazing division of labor. Some are assigned to the nursery; some stand guard to ward off intruders; some provide air conditioning—beating their wings to produce heat in the winter and to provide a cool air flow in the summer. Some attend strictly to the needs of the queen and others have the task of cleaning. At some time, nearly all bees are involved in bringing home the nectar.

Lessons from the Bee

Be a worker. A bee may be sort of a workaholic, but if we would each do our part and productively help others, as they do, we would be blessed!

Be sweet. Bees rather reluctantly give up their honey. How wonderful it is when we willingly spread joy, beauty, pleasantness, and sweetness to those around us.

CAMEL: PREPARED FOR STORMS

It is easier for a camel to go through the eye of the needle than for someone who is rich to enter the kingdom of God . . . For mortals it is impossible, but not for God; for God all things are possible (Mark 10:25, 27 NRSV).

No animal is better prepared for the devastating storms of the desert than the camel. Our scripture verse suggests the storm of difficulty some have in being true disciples, but with God all things are possible.

Scientists tell us that the camel has been man's servant for longer than any other creature. Not only is it capable of providing transportation in the nearly impossible desert terrain, but it also provides milk, cheese, hair for blankets, and texts, and even meat. Mark 1:6 speaks of John the Baptist as clothed with camel's hair. In transportation of goods, the camel can carry as much as 1,000 pounds.

God the Creator did a masterful job in preparing the camel for the desert. The eyes are protected by over-hanging lids and long lashes which shield it from the intense sun. The nostrils can be closed tight against driving sand of the storms. The camel's upper lip can reach out for shrubs, and its very strong teeth can chew almost anything. If no other food is around it can eat leather, blankets, bones, or whole fish. It will even drink salty water. Nothing seems to give it indigestion. An added feature, its large two-toed feet are especially cushioned for walking on the sand.

We have assumed that the Wise Men bringing their gifts to Jesus traveled by camel, but the Bible doesn't state that. Camels might indicate great wealth; Job after his suffering was blessed with 6,000 camels.

Lessons from the Camel

Meet the storms on your knees. The camel is not known for its obedience or intelligence, except when it faces a storm. When the wind begins to blow strong enough to blow sand, the camel drops to its knees, closes its nostrils, stretches out its neck, and remains motionless until the storm has passed, thus protecting itself and its rider.

Carry your burdens patiently. Although stubborn, once loaded and started the camel will patiently carry its load great distances. Often our burdens seem more than we can bear. With God's help the load can be mastered, perhaps even turned into a cross-crown of glory (Mark 8:34–37).

PALM TREE: THE RIGHTEOUS SHALL FLOURISH

The righteous shall flourish like the palm tree (Psalm 92:12 KJV).

The palm tree plays a very prominent part in the plants of the Bible. Exodus 15:27 is the first place where the palm tree is used. This is where Moses and the Israelites are traveling through the wilderness, and an oasis is found: "Next they came to Elim, where there were twelve springs and seventy palm trees; there they camped by the water."

Palm trees are distinct in an oasis. When traveling through a desert area, discovering a palm tree in the distance means water, a pressing necessity, is near. Thousands of Israelites were with Moses and desperate for water. At Elim they found water amid the palm trees.

Many naturalists agree that the palm is the most remarkable of all trees. One remarkable quality is its ability to withstand storms. A hurricane may blow a palm tree over, but from its prostrate position, it will again lift its head, and the growing top will become upright. Also remarkable is that the palm tree can withstand fire without being destroyed. Instead of having a layer of fragile bark like most trees, the growth is from within. A complete outer layer of bark could be removed, and the tree would not be destroyed. The palm tree's height is a remarkable feature, with some trees reaching 100 feet in height.

Virtually all human needs can be met in the amazing palm tree. The date palm, referred to in the Bible, can provide food, shelter, and clothing. This tree provides more agricultural wealth and nutritional food per acre than perhaps any other tree. Palm branches can be used as a building material, and palm leaves can be used for clothing. Also, they are satisfactory for use as fuel for a fire. The Palmyra palm tree of India has about 800 different uses. Worldwide there are more than 1,500 different kinds of palms. In Bible usage, the palm tree is referred to 32 times.

Another unusual quality of the palm tree is its growth point, known as the terminal bud. It is at the very top of the tree, from which growth takes place. If the terminal bud is not disturbed, almost nothing can destroy the tree. Fire can burn around it, a storm can blow it over, and it will continue to flourish. But if the bud is destroyed, the tree dies. Regrettably, the terminal bud is considered a delicacy called palm cabbage. In some nations, it is harvested to eat, thus destroying the tree.

Palm Sunday is a significant day in the Christian year. In celebration of Jesus entering Jerusalem, palm branches were cut from nearby palm trees and waved in his honor or placed on the ground before him. Palm branches were an accepted tribute for royalty.

Lessons from the Palm Tree

The righteous will flourish like palm trees; they will grow like the cedars of Lebanon. They are like trees planted in the house of the Lord, that flourish in the Temple of our God, that still bear fruit in old age and are always green and strong (Psalm 92:12–14 TEV).

We could have the terminal bud symbolize our living relationship with God. Keep that relationship active and growing. Even if the storms and fires come, we will endure. If we destroy our relationship with God, all that is valuable in life is destroyed.

The Meaning of Suffering

David Belgum

The word "suffering" has this linguistic background. The Latin derivation implies being under a burden, suf (sub) + fer (to bear). To bear up under. Pain is hard to bear. Sufferers sometimes say, "It is my cross to bear." It is oppressive, makes one feel like a victim. Yes, it is heavy and burdensome.

The Greek word for suffering, "pathos," has enriched our language. The College of Medicine has a major department studying the pathology of patients, their diseases, malfunctions, deformities and suffering. As we leave the room of a dying patient, someone will remark how pathetic the emaciated child looks. It is considered a virtue to have sympathy with a sufferer. Counselors have more recently been encouraged to enter even more fully into the client's experience with empathy.

Suffering bears so many faces and diverse manifestations that it is hard to know where to begin in discussing it or analyzing it. It may even seem indecent to try to be objective about so subjective an experience. Yet in our calmer moments we do know that before we can deal with a situation effectively, or as usefully as possible, it is helpful to try to understand what we are up against. In the healing arts, diagnosis comes before treatment. Knowing the problem comes before seeking an answer or solution. And, of course, sometimes there is no solution. There certainly is much suffering that is incurable. There may be some ameliorating help and support, but no cure. Yet when we cannot cure, we may still be privileged to care.

For our purpose we shall focus on three types of suffering. Physical pain, mental distress, and social discord. Pain of the body is so immediate and obvious that it is a good place to begin our discussion. Mental distress is less visible as it relates to the psyche, the interior world of our private thoughts. Others do not know it unless we reveal it by self-disclosure. Social suffering is elusive because it is often taken for granted or even culturally sanctioned, e.g., group discrimination or stigma.

PHYSICAL PAIN

About fifty years ago at the University of Minnesota, our psychology text-book had a clever diagram showing how pain messages were sent from one outlying point to the brain. A series of telegraph poles and wires ran from the stubbed toe up the leg to the bottom of the spinal cord and thence to the brain. Little lightening type flashes ran along the wire to indicate the electrical pulses. This looked similar to a picture of telegraph poles erected along the Missouri River in western Iowa. A person wanting to send a message from Sioux City to Omaha would hand the message to the telegraph operator in the Sioux City office but then to make sure it got prompt attention he would bribe the operator with a shot or two of whiskey. Then it would be transferred quickly to the wire and flashed (the electric impulse) to Denver. From there it would be picked up by another pony express rider who would rush it up past Thalamus Ridge to Cerebral Mountain Peak, the headquarters. The General would have to decide how to respond. There's no time to lose. No sooner have I completed this new, revised illustration than I realize any use of telegraph wire will be inadequate. Maybe it is more like a net with many alternate routes of transmission.

Dr. Kerr wrote *The Pain Book* from the perspective of a neuroanatomist at Mayo Clinic. It blows my mind to discover how much more complex our central nervous message system is than the one I described in the previous paragraph:

> It is probable, therefore, that there are more than 100 billion neurons in the entire human nervous system, a prodigious and totally incomprehensible figure . . . neurons communicate with each other by means of an axon. This extremely slender filament, on reaching its target, usually breaks up into a number of fine terminal branches, each of which ends with a tiny bulbous swelling known as a bouton, or end bulb.[1]

Across this infinitesimal gap, or synapse, the pain message is passed along by a neurochemical transmitter, one of several chemical agents I won't even try to name (hence my reference to a couple of shots of whiskey in my revised diagram above). Kerr claims that delicate instrumentation has measured the speed of these message transmissions in certain types of nerves at 260 miles per hour. It can be measured in milliseconds (1,000th of a second).

Measuring the size of these tiny nerve fibers is equally amazing. The book shows cross sections of fibers magnified by 24,000 times. At that rate a human hair would appear to be almost five feet in diameter.[2]

One of the functions of this intricate complex of neural message systems is to alert us to trouble and danger. Just the messages plain and simple are not worth much until they are decoded and interpreted. Somewhere in the brain a decision is made: "Remove your hand from that red hot stove burner, and I mean RIGHT NOW!!" Thus physical pain is very useful in protecting the whole self from danger and further injury. It is also remarkably educational. We learn not to repeat the "hand on the red hot burner sequence."

As in any efficient organization, delegation of authority and responsibility is present in the nervous system. It comes in three levels. First, a simple response can be obtained directly from the spinal column, such as withdrawal from a painful stimulus, without having to go all the way to the brain. Secondly, the cortex registers more precise information such as the type of pain. Third, in the upper brain stem there is a general alerting system, which arouses the total organism to the danger and urges it to react. Hence, even in this very automatic and basic neural system there is a quick interpretation of the meaning of the pain message. (Conversation with Dr. Brigitte Bendixon, Department of Neurology, University of Iowa Hospitals and Clinics.)

Unfortunately, we don't have the benefit of pain when we need it sometimes. Wouldn't it be wonderful if a person were struck with acute and excruciating pain upon drinking the third glass of beer at one sitting. Or if a person smoked more than one cigarette a day, he developed life-threatening and painful shortness of breath. Unfortunately the person must smoke two packs a day for twenty years before he ends up in the intensive care unit with a pair of green nasal prongs in his nose. Sometimes that Serpent who used to live in the Garden if Eden deceives us by camouflaging the danger as pleasant and beneficial. If consequences of danger are delayed, the educational impact is lost.

Since physical pain is so organically based and tissue related, we are inclined to think that pain is pain. X amount of stimulus results in Y amount of response. Apparently it is not that simple. David Morris in his book, *The Culture of Pain*, illustrates the social and ethnic and circumstantial variables that give pain different meanings in different situations.[3] Two ancient Greek city states differed remarkably in this regard. The Spartans were stoical and trained from childhood on to endure physical hardship without complaint. They were hardy soldiers. The Athenians, on the other hand, maybe because they were intellectual effete snobs, did not place much store by such values and were not known for hardiness. Kerr cites two extreme cases in our time. "The gap that separates the response of a Cossack who allows his foot to be amputated with apparent complete indifference to pain from that of a person who cries out in anguish when pricked with a sharp hypodermic needle is evidently enormous."[4]

Lieutenant Colonel Henry K. Beecher made these observations from his experience in World War II. He speculated that the reason seventy-five percent of the wounded soldiers refused pain medication was due to the significance or meaning of their wounds.

> . . . consider the position of the soldier: his wound suddenly releases him from an exceedingly dangerous environment, one filled with fatigue, discomfort, anxiety, fear, and real danger of death, and gives him a ticket to the safety of the hospital. His troubles are about over . . . On the other hand, the civilian's accident marks the beginning of disaster for him.[5]

This immediate painlessness may be followed later on by a "flood of grief and fear . . . His arm is injured—will he lose it? There is blood around his genitals—will he be impotent? That wound in his chest—is he going to die? The pain cannot be separated from the personal questions and social meaning it inescapably evokes."[6]

There can also be a powerful religious meaning ascribed to the pain and to the injury or disease causing the pain. "What have I done that God is punishing me so severely?" Pain comes from the Latin poene, which means literally penalty or punishment. There is an ancient tradition going back to the book of Job called the doctrine of retribution:

> Think now, who that was innocent ever perished?
> Or where were the upright cut off?
> As I have seen those who plow iniquity
> And sow trouble reap the same.
> By the breath of God they perish
> And by the blast of his anger they are consumed. (Job 4:7–8)

The message of the judgmental counselor, Eliphaz, is clear: "You, Job, must have sinned mightily since the blast of God's anger has caused you so much suffering, the death of your children and now these awful boils all over your miserable body." The plaintive cry goes up from many a modern hospital bed: "Why did this happen to me?" It is a cry searching for some meaning in one's suffering, in one's pain.

When Paterson studied how families were dealing with the distress of having a cerebral palsied child, several options of interpretation were offered.[7] The parents opted for "punishment" over "meaninglessness." It appears that even such a negative and oppressive concept was preferable to meaninglessness. How could such a distressing experience, likely the most stressful event in their married life, have no purpose, no meaning at all?

Meanwhile the scientific/medical community is devoted to objectivity and explanations about the "how" of disease, pain and suffering, not the "why". So patients are left to surmise this or that concerning the cause of their pain. Sometimes patients remember acts committed by them years ago for which they should justly have been punished, but they got by with it temporarily because no one else knew about it. But God has a long memory and finally gets around to meting out justice, or so goes the retribution theory.

Rabbi Kushner, has made an excellent contribution to the above dilemma in his book, *When Bad Things Happen To Good People*.[8] He lifts the discussion out of the rut of retribution theory with the assumption that the "why" question is usually almost impossible to answer anyway. Oh, there are instances when the cause and effect is clearly moral as in such cases as the vice of gluttony leading to health damaging obesity, when escape from moral responsibility leads to devastating drug addiction, etc. But in so many cases the search for "why" causes is futile. Kushner suggests we change the questions to a more fruitful one, which is also on a higher spiritual plane. "Now that this has happened to me, what will my response be?" Whereas the retribution approach often leads to endless self -castigation, Kushner's question focuses on "response" or responsibility. How can I make use of pain, suffering or disability in some constructive way: maybe joining a support group or substituting some positive goal or attitude for the lack of self-esteem which has plagued me thus far. This provides a realistic and legitimate alternative to self pity, hostility and bitterness, which is our temptation in the face of unconquerable adversity. Maybe instead of focusing on what I have lost, I can dwell on what I have left. After all, I am still a child of God and created in His image. Some have even written their story as a testimony and encouragement to other sufferers. Worthwhile meaning can replace hopeless despair.

Lest you think the previous paragraph smacks of Pollyannaism, let me hasten to remind you that we said earlier that sometimes there is no solution. There may be only unmitigated tragedy. One well wisher glibly tried to comfort a patient in excruciating circumstances thus: "Cheer up; things could be worse." So, he cheered up and sure enough, things got worse.

Paterson helpfully describes three kinds of pain, each with its own characteristics and potential and meaning.[9] They are acute, chronic and terminal. Acute pain, like the message to remove your hand from the red hot burner, conveys an accurate and very useful message; and there is often something that can be done about it: Visit your dentist, remove the sliver or change some destructive behavior. Even with proper medication and supportive counseling the arthritic pain may continue long after the message, "You're in trouble," has been heard loud and clear. In terminal pain, "sometimes the pain seems to become a focus for all the distress the person feels over dying—fear, anger, sadness, loneliness, shame, and guilt—as though it were easier to cope with one part of the process than with the whole."[10]

Physical pain is being studied more intensively of late, There is now the International Association for the Study of Pain. Major hospitals have set up pain clinics with an interdisciplinary approach drawing upon the fields of medicine, neurology, surgery, pharmacology, physical therapy, nursing, social work and chaplaincy, to name a few.[11] This is because physical pain is multifaceted. I see now that I was naïve in listing the three parts in this paper; physical pain, emotional distress, and social discord with the assumption that I was moving from the specific and simple to the more general and complex. I now see that physical pain is inextricably infiltrated with psychological, social and spiritual factors and meanings.

All health care givers, including clergy, need to be sensitive to the many nuances and meanings of pain and suffering of patients and counselees. If we listen carefully maybe they will share what their pain means to them; and then we can go on from there to use our resources and time appropriately.

MENTAL DISTRESS

The kind of mental process I am referring to here is that private and interior world to which we communicate mostly with our own selves. It involves depression, brooding, reflecting on our own low self-esteem and feeling bad about it. There are many private, painful sorrows that are not shared with others, may not even originate from the outside. It is our own way of thinking about ourselves and our situation, the meaning of our own experiences, those emotions, feelings and thoughts which are our very own.

The inferiority complex is a good case in point. You may have been in a class of thirty junior high students with your grades and all else indicating you are a perfectly normal or, at least, average person. Yet within you may have been a gnawing insecurity, hesitation to attempt a task for fear of failure, stage fright, or passive quietness, the kind that you hope will make you so inconspicuous that no one will notice you. One person might describe it as loneliness, another as shame. Embarrassment can be a painful experience even while you are putting up a fairly good front so that no one else shares your sad experience. This can be a kind of invisible mental distress. Sometimes our body language gives us away, we blush, avert our gaze or jam our fists deep into our trouser pockets and give ourselves away. But it was because we were trying hard to keep our inner thoughts and feelings secret. Shame means it is not alright to be who you are, Perhaps a person (you) has seriously harmed his neighbor by committing acts which may have gone unnoticed in society, but inwardly your conscience convicts you and you suffer mentally, psychologically. When you finally confess to a priest or counselor, you may say, "For two years I've been just sick over this mess." Sometimes such a one becomes deeply depressed and says to the self, "You don't deserve happiness, you deserve the misery you have brought upon yourself." Here again is the retribution doctrine, but you don't need anyone else to tell you — you know it all too well, for "the still small voice" has told you.

The list of negative emotions within us can be long indeed and it seems that most of them have been spewed out upon the stage or spread across the TV screen: anger, sorrow, self pity, jealousy, slavery to addiction, lust, greed, burning resentments, fear, doubts, pessimism, varieties of sadness, and a sense of impending doom. Just as the masochist seems to need to want physical pain for some unconscious dynamic, folks with the above ruminations seem to have gotten into a rut of negative thinking in which these festering mental sores keep on being re-infected and exacerbated. Saint Paul writes to the Galations about such "works of the flesh." Paul uses the Greek term sarx, flesh, not soma, body (see 5:19–23). Meanwhile, he favors the power of positive thinking: "But the fruit of the Spirit is love, joy, peace, long-suffering, gentleness, goodness, faith, meekness, temperance; against such there is no law." And such thought and attitudes also do not cause mental suffering. It almost sounds like they could be the medicinal antidote some people need, like an antibiotic that gets rid of pesky germs.

Reason and Emotion in Psychotherapy was Albert Ellis' first textbook presenting "rational-emotive therapy."[12] Ellis asserted that what goes on in one's mind as far as ascribing meaning to a given event is prior to the emotion (of fear, anger, etc.). Let us say that your lawn mower won't start some summer day when your grass is already far too long. Anger is not your first experience. First you think, "How unfair the world is. I don't deserve such tough luck. I decided to make myself angry about this awful injustice." Only then do you kick the lawn mower. You were equally free to say to yourself, "I guess I'd better take this lawn mower down to the shop and see if the mechanic can get it started." In the latter case it is not a federal case after all, just an inactive lawn mower. Ellis makes a good case for paying attention to the mental dynamics that go on within ourselves. Maybe we do not need to generate as much mental distress as we sometimes create. And it might be cheaper than Tylenol or aspirin.

A poignant case in point is that of the fugitive, Katherine Ann Power, who was sentenced for her part involving the death of Boston police officer, Walter Schroeder. While eating breakfast a few days ago, I saw her on the TV news making this statement: "I cannot possibly say how sorry I am for what happened." After the shooting she had moved to the Pacific coast. Even her husband of fourteen years knew nothing of her inner turmoil. Even during the numerous shared meals, private conversations and even during sexual intercourse (for which the Hebrew Bible uses the term "to know") this knowledge did not slip out in an unguarded moment. It must have seemed like being in a psychological solitary confinement cell. Yes, mental distress. How emotions must have been mingled with behavior, feelings of fear of being apprehended, some rationalization of how crimes of theft and murder were in a "good cause", the Vietnam anti-war protest movement, the moral dilemma of turning oneself in after having, after all, "earned" a respectable place in society once again, back and forth, back and forth, the struggle, the mental pain—all of it a completely private and interior experience.

Meanwhile, Ms. Power's psychotherapist maintains that her client is clinically depressed, maybe due to chemical imbalance. More and more psychiatrists and neurologists are stressing the organic factor in mental states, the conditioning influence of genetic traits, the intoxicating effects of chemicals, especially chemical imbalance, tangled or misaligned nerves, traumatic injuries, glands and organs gone bonkers, etc. The therapist said that clinical depression ran in Ms. Power's family.

Remember in our introduction how I had sought such a logical progression from the physical, bodily, organic level of suffering on up to the more intangible, psychological, or even spiritual level of mental distress, then finally arriving at the most generic, social (way out there) kind of suffering. Personality is no longer that simple; psychosomatic understandings no longer allow us that luxury. Just as mental states can influence our perception and interpretation of physical pain, so organic factors are a substrate for our thoughts, feelings, emotions and mental frame of mind. There would be no conscious experience, psychological, subconscious or verbal, without those tiny nerve endings described above, without the brain with its interlocking and intercommunicating lobes and folds. Influence goes in both directions. That is why it is a fallacy to over-spiritualize our life's experiences, or, on the other hand, to settle for a minimalist materialism, which may discount such factors as beliefs, values, and psychological motivations. Saint Paul said that the person is made up of many members: the eye, the ear, the hand, etc. These are all gifts of creation and are all needed to make up the whole body. Paul says," ... there are varieties of gifts, but the same Spirit ... for the common good."[13] I guess our assignment is to integrate all facets so our personality and character can deal with whatever life offers us whether joy or sorrow. We must consider success of failure, riches or poverty, good health or physical distress, whatever in the end might affect our Psyche. Hard to explain but I think you know what I mean.

SOCIAL DISCORD

Social experiences are those related to other persons, often in groups. We have interactions with social clubs, church choir, other workers in factory or office jobs, recreational groups like bowling leagues, institutions whether educational, financial or governmental. We do not live in a vacuum; that is for sure. In so many ways we are interdependent. We belong to groups for different reasons, to meet different needs; and sometimes these needs are in conflict or mutually exclusive. Then amidst the tensions, arguments, fights and lawsuits, we find ourselves in turmoil, which I choose to call social suffering. There has been no injury to your body, but there are scars on your soul. Your pride may be wounded, your feelings hurt. This is different from purely mental distress because it is not so private. The struggle is external as well as internal. It may even have been reported in the daily newspaper. It influences your interpersonal relationships. Someone you always thought you could count on as a trusted friend now no longer associates with you because you are "on the wrong side," whether the conflict be over school bussing, abortion rights, fair housing or sexism. If you were offered an option, you might even choose a broken leg or a broken heart rather than this broken relationship, i.e., if you had the choice. So often whatever our current distress or pain or suffering is, it seems worse than many other problems; maybe because it is mine and it is now.

Maybe there are as many social synapses in our lives as there are between those tiny nerve endings. How often we have said, "He/she really gets on my nerves." You, a quiet introvert, decided not to invite your old classmate, who is such a bombastic extrovert, to your daughter's wedding. Well, count on getting one fewer Christmas cards next winter. Who knows how much distress it might cause one, but at least it is on the negative side. It would have been nice if the issue had not arisen.

We do not always have control over painful issues arising. A black surgeon, who can easily afford to buy the new house on Overlook Drive with a lovely pond at the lower end of a spacious yard, may run into racial prejudice. This was especially true when Ku Klux Klan was stronger than the U.S. Constitution. Many racial barriers have been removed with legislation, civil rights marches and other forces of change and accommodation. Sometimes as old conflicts fade into the background, new challenges and tensions emerge. It may be utopian to hope that some day all conflict will cease. In the real world this hope is not yet realized. In the Balkans, latent social conflict, which lay dormant for seventy years under the heel of Big Brother, has now burst into warfare since the restraints have been lifted.

One out of every two marriages today is expected to end in divorce; and even when the separation is fairly amicable, there is grief work to tend to without the social support of a funeral like in the case of separation by death. And certainly in families which may be judged successful and very functional in every way, there are tensions as children struggle through their adolescent grasp for independence and increasing autonomy. In fact, if a child's growth toward mature adulthood is totally devoid of struggle, that person is deprived of important meaning. You mean my growing up is of no consequence, does not cause a ripple in the family? I thought I was more important than that. That is like entering a tennis tournament and having all the potential opponents forfeit, and then getting the trophy, never having played a match. We must not confuse struggle and hard work with suffering. Healthy fatigue after accomplishing a hard day's work is not only natural but good for us; it can provide us with a pleasant feeling of satisfaction and self esteem.

Social disgrace can drive a person to distraction and even despair. Consider the student in junior high, who lived in a town so gung ho for football that anyone not enthusiastic about the game nor trying out for the team was guilty of treason and considered a worthless wimp. The lad became so down on himself that his physician and counselor both thought he was in danger of committing suicide. Thus the cycle would have been complete: social suffering leading to mental misery. In this case the student transferred to a private school in another community and is now thriving. This puts the lie to the old adage: "Sticks and stone can break my bones, but words can never hurt me."

Persons who "deviate from the norm" face social pressure and rejection. Simmons discovered that a large variety of things or persons are declared deviant by someone or another. Of the 180 subjects in his survey, they listed 252 distinct acts and persons as deviant. Here are a few of the items listed as deviant:

Homosexuals, prostitutes, drug addicts, criminals, liars, career women, Democrats, atheists, Christians, suburbanites, the retired, young folks, bearded men, artists, priests, conservatives, divorcees, know-it-all professors.[14]

In other words, I am the norm and anyone who differs from me is a deviant. This study highlighted how irrational and whimsical the process of stigmatizing various categories of persons is. Yet for the object of such judgmentalism, the social sugaring consists in being put down, depersonalized, insulted and made a scapegoat. It often means not only rejection, but also exclusion from some social group or activity because of being a "second class citizen". From Simmons' list we see how pervasive such prejudice is. Practically everyone has the golden opportunity of being snubbed and abused socially whether for being too short or too tall, too rich or too poor, for stuttering, limping, forgetting, for being boorish or a social snob. Naturally, some persons take these jobs more seriously than others; but it is likely that in any given category there are those who take such depreciation seriously, personally and painfully. We could call it social suffering.

We now understand that spousal or child abuse is not limited to assault and battery but can be equally painful when it takes the form of psychological abuse, ridicule, or in many other ways resulting in the victim's (usually a child) "Failure to thrive." The symptoms of child abuse are not limited to bruises and fractured bones, but can include nightmares, fear of doom, enuresis, loss of appetite, physical symptoms, inability to concentrate at school, inability to trust others, lack of self confidence, shame, guilt, ("I must be a really bad boy to make my father this angry"), etc. The reason I classify this with social suffering is that it is not merely a matter of one's inward thoughts and feelings, but involves interpersonal and social relations (or should we say anti-social relations?).

There are today increasing legal protections for victims of abuse: safe shelters for battered wives, foster care for abused children, cease and desist court orders, etc. Fortunately these efforts have greatly reduced social suffering.

The "victim' is not solely dependent upon outside help to deal with social suffering. A person can develop interior attitudes and personal behaviors that can also reduce the suffering. When "Fatso" is ridiculed on the playground, the boy can chime in and say, "Yeah, that's me alright; I'd make a great goalie on your hockey team, fill the whole net." Suddenly it is not rewarding to tease the boy. Defensiveness just makes the matter worse. It is like a flock of chickens where one hen has been injured and bleeding. The others peck at the sore and pick on the poor thing till it bleeds to death. Some parents help their child to "consider the source" and thus take some of the power away from the bully or teaser or ridiculer. Sometimes professional therapy, like in a speech clinic, rehabilitation clinic, or counseling service, can assist the person feel less of a victim and put the name calling into proper perspective.

Social relations can be a two-edged sword. The previous discussion has focused on the negative, when social suffering results. We also need social interaction. "Seeing ourselves as others see us" keeps us in touch with reality. As we see ourselves reflected in the pupils of the eyeballs of others, like those multiple mirrors in the clothing stores, we see ourselves in perspective. We need to be open to the suggestions, evaluations and criticism of others, at least hear them and give them considered attention. Many have grown and matured by such openness. But it is our responsibility to distinguish between constructive and destructive input from others. We are free to reject the negative or to embrace it as social suffering, a kind of socio-masochism.

SPIRITUAL RESOURCES FOR SUFFERERS

If one's religion is a positive resource, there are many biblical supports for Ego integrity and wholesome self regard. According to Genesis, we humans are created in the image of God. As one wag put it bluntly, "God does not create junk."

> When I look at your heavens, the work of your fingers
> What are human beings that you are mindful of them
> Yet you have made them a little lower than the angels
> And crowned them with glory and honor. (Psalm 8:3,4,5)

Jesus admonished his disciples to hold their head up:

> Are not two sparrows sold for a penny?
> Yet not one of them will fall to the ground without your Father's will.
> But even the hairs of your head are all numbered
> Fear not, therefore, you are of more
> Value than many sparrows. (Matt. 10:29–31)

This is all good news for victims of social suffering, the put downs that tempt a person to self depreciation at the suggestion of others. The grace of God means the unlimited acceptance by our Creator in spite of this or that peculiarity, defect or fault.

If the opposite of pain is pleasure, that does not mean that pleasure is to be sought at any price. Great saints and heroic persons have accepted pain rather than forsake their God, their values or their beliefs, but martyrdom was the inevitable consequence for some, such as Dietrich Bonhoeffer, Martin Luther King, Jr., Mahatma Gandhi, to name a few. Jesus admonished, "Fear not those who kill the body but cannot kill the soul . . . " (Matt. 20:28)

The suffering servant is a profound theme in scripture. Saint Paul suffered persecution but thought it was worth it. "I consider that the sufferings of this present time are not worth comparing with the glory about to be revealed to us." (Romans 8:18)

The body of Jesus hanging on the cross is for many the epitome of suffering: a combination of physical pain, mental distress and social suffering. Catholic believers are urged to merge their sufferings with those of Jesus and somehow offer them up to God. This gives ultimate meaning to their suffering and pains. It can be more than a hopeless resignation: it can be a conscious and deliberate commitment. Many a petitioner includes somewhere in the prayer, "If it be Thy will."

The beloved poet/pastor of Iceland, Hallgrimur Petursson, wrote *Hymns of the Passion* and said this in a verse about the verbal abuse and shame heaped upon Jesus on the cross:

> The world's abuse I often meet
> And weep in my affliction
> But find with Thee a safe retreat
> Healing and benediction.
> Beneath Thy cross I take my stand
> The floods of scorn ignoring
> Happy and safe in Thy dear hand
> My heart Thy grace adoring[15]

I have known dying patients whose pains cannot be cured, but who have found great comfort in a caring God as described in Deuteronomy 33:27, "The eternal God is your dwelling place, and underneath are the everlasting arms."

CONCLUSION

The search for meaning is a uniquely human experience.[16] It places us on a higher level than when we just drift along unquestioningly following the path of least resistance. Meaning of suffering is not inherent in the suffering, whether it be of the physical, mental or social type. We must find the meaning, create a meaning, ask ourselves, "What does this mean for me?" We grow and heal in the very process of searching for the meaning of suffering, our own or that or others.

NOTES

1. Frederick W.L. err, *The Brain Book*. Englewood Cliffs, New Jersey: Prentice Hall, 1981, pp. 16–17.

2. Ibid. Chapter 2, "Nerves, the Brain, and Pain," provides even more fascinating detailed information about the neural information system and it function.

3. David B. Morris, *The Culture of Pain*, Berkeley, California: University of California Press, 1993, Chapter 2, "The Meaning of Pain."

4. Kerr, *op.cit.* p.10.

5. Henry K. Beecher, "Pain in Men Wounded in Battle," *The Bulletin of the U.S. Army Medical Department*, April 1946, p. 448. See also his "Relationship of Significance of Wound to the Pain Experience," *J.A.M.A.*, 161 (1956). ½ 1609–1613.

6. Morris, *op.cit.,* p.43.

7. George W. Paterson, "An Exploratory Study of the Role of Religion Among Families with a Cerebral Palsied Child." PhD dissertation, University of Iowa, 1969.

8. Harold Kushner, *When Bad Things Happen To Good People.* New York: Schocken Books, 1981.

9. George W. Paterson, "The Pastoral Care of Persons in Pain, " *Journal of Religion and Aging* Vol. I (1), Fall 1984.

10. Ibid p. 23.

11. Other references dealing with pain are the following: Michael R. Bond, *Pain, Its Nature Analysis and Treatment,* Edinburgh: Churchill Livingston, 1984, Ben E. Benjamin, *Listen to Your Pain, The Active Person's Guide to Understanding, Identifying and Treating Pain and Injury,* New York: The Viking Press, 1984 . C. Norman Shealy, *The Pain Game.* California, Celestial Arts, 1976. Bill Moyers, *Healing and the Mind,* New York: Doubleday, 1993. Ronald Melzack, "The Perception of Pain. *Scientific American* Volume 204, No. 2 February, 1961, pp. 41–49.

12. Albert Ellis, *Reason and Emotion in Psychotherapy,* Secaucus, New Jersey: Citadel 1977 (paperback edition).

13. See all of chapter 12: I Corinthians, for the context of these brief phrases.

14. J.L. Simmons, *Deviants* The Glendessary Press (N.P.) 1969, p. 3 See also Erving Goffman's pioneering work, *Stigma: Notes On Management of Spoiled Identity.*Englewood Cliffs, New Jersey: Prentice Hall, 1963. David Belgum, *What Can I Do About the Part of Me I Don't Like?* Minneapolis, Minnesota: Augsburg Publishing House, 1974. This book grew out of the author's own wrestling with the stigma associated with stuttering as a negative social experience.

15. Hallgrimur Petersson, *Hymns of the Passion: Meditations on the Passion of Christ* (Translated by Arthur Charles Cook) Reykjavik, Iceland: Hallgrims Church, 1978 p. 163 (First Icelandic edition, 1666).

16. Viktor E. Frankl, *The Unheard Cry for Meaning* New York: Simon and Schuster, 1978. He maintains that searching for meaning is therapeutic as well as useful for personal growth.

Contributors

MEMBERS OF WRITERS GROUP

Otto Bauer is a retired university administrator.

David Belgum was an emeritus professor of Religion and Medicine at the University of Iowa.

Stanley Elder is a retired farmer/agri-businessman.

David Good is a retired judge of the 6th Judicial District Court of Iowa.

Sam Hahn is a retired minister of the United Methodist Church.

Pat Healy is a former art teacher in the public schools.

Bill Lyons taught secondary English and served as a language arts coordinator in the Iowa City, Iowa, Community School District.

Caryl Lyons is a teacher of English as a Second Language and a test developer for college entrance exams.

Bob McCown is a retired librarian of the University of Iowa Libraries.

Earl Rose is a retired professor of Pathology at the University of Iowa.